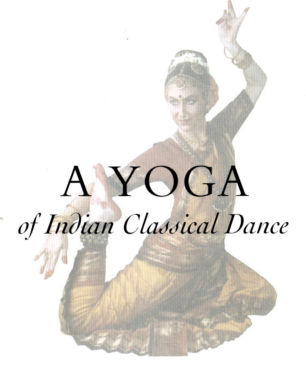

A YOGA
of Indian Classical Dance

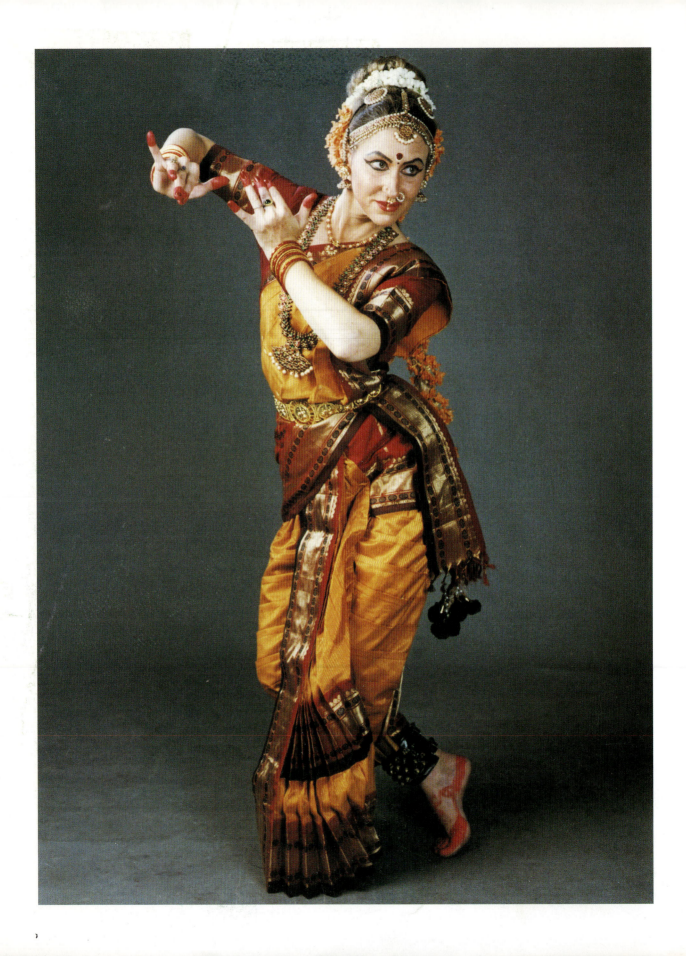

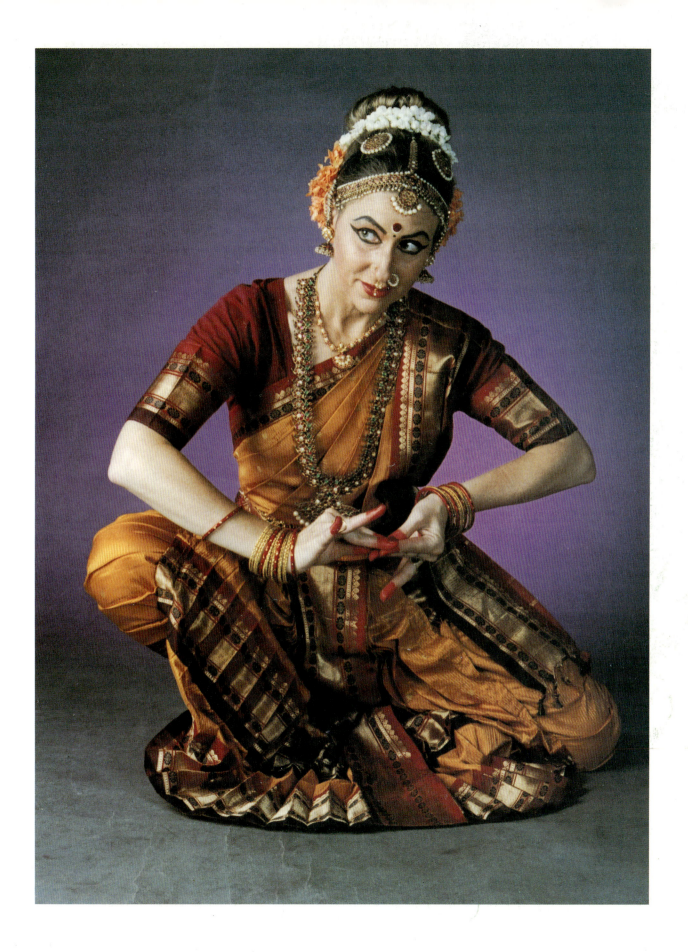

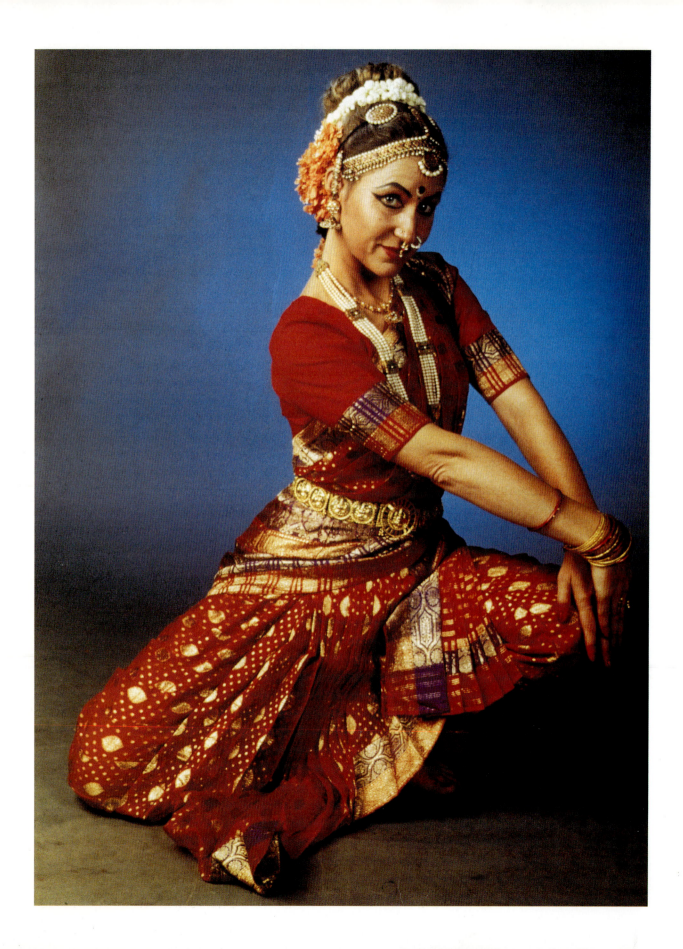

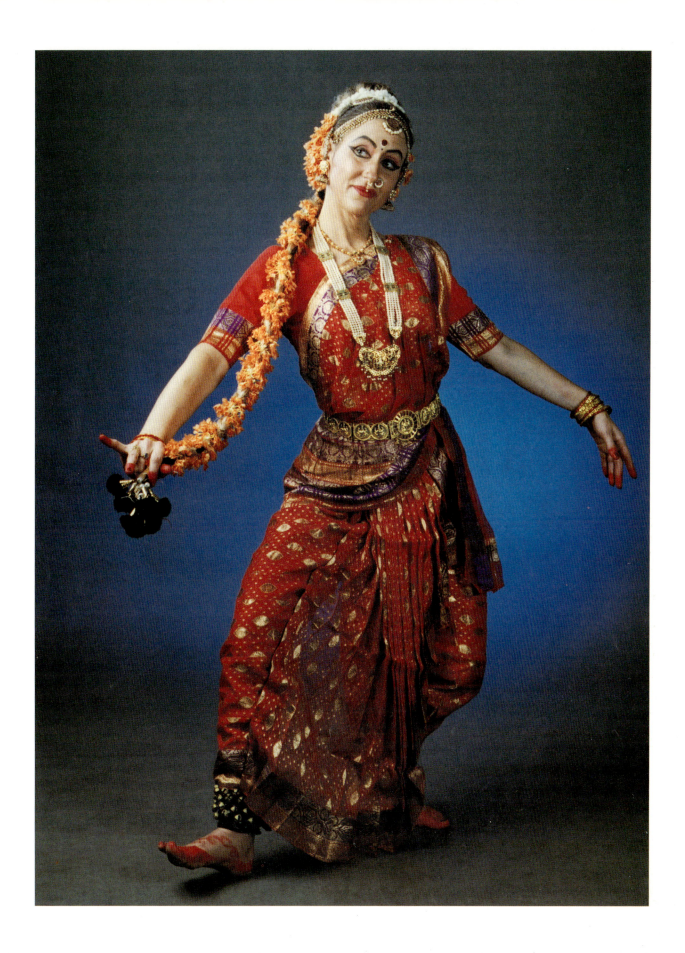

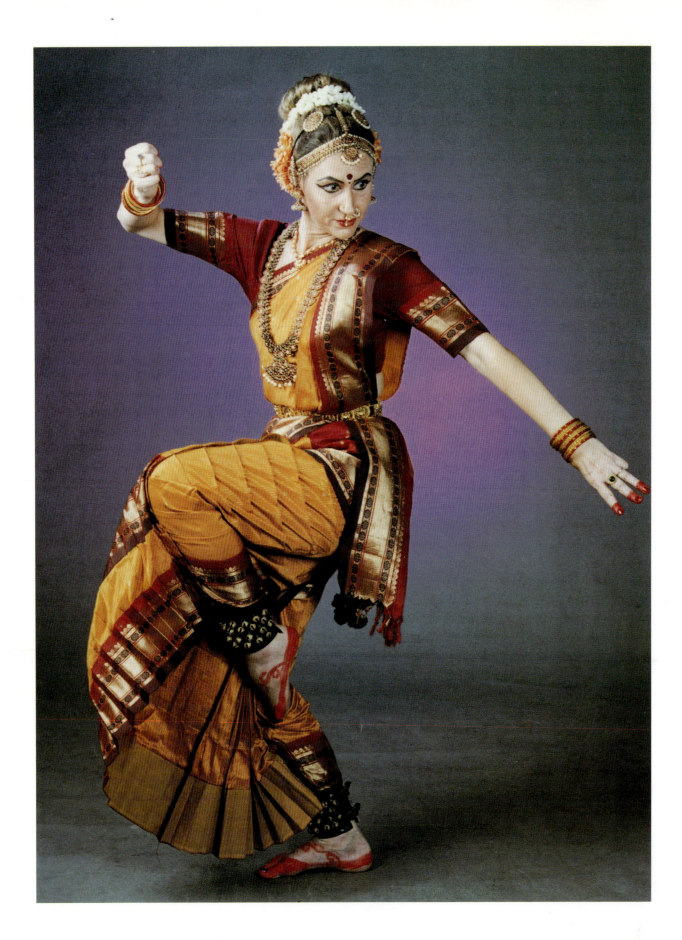

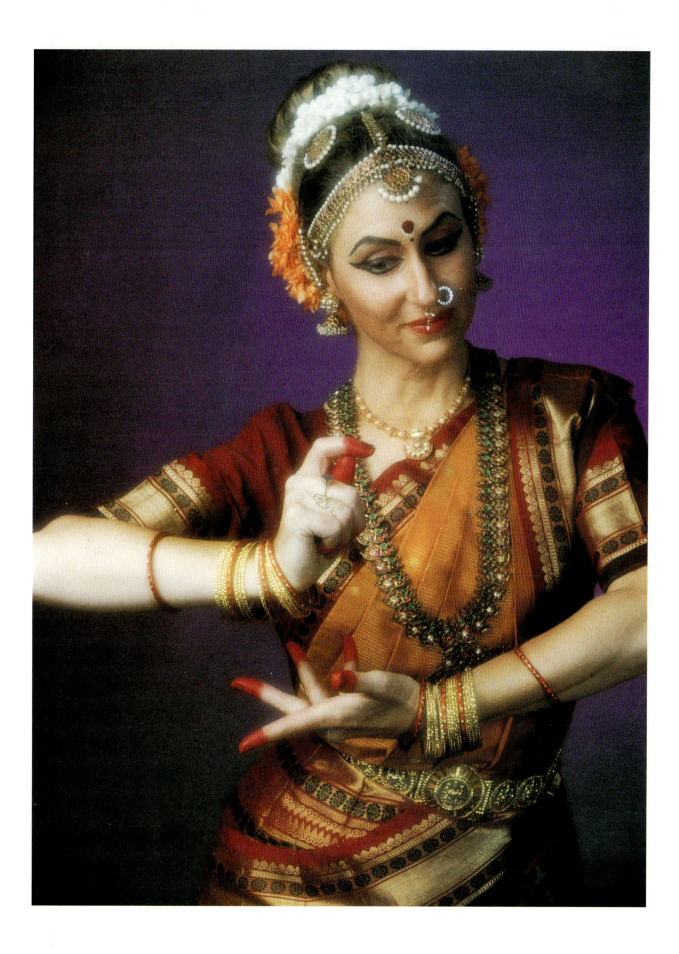

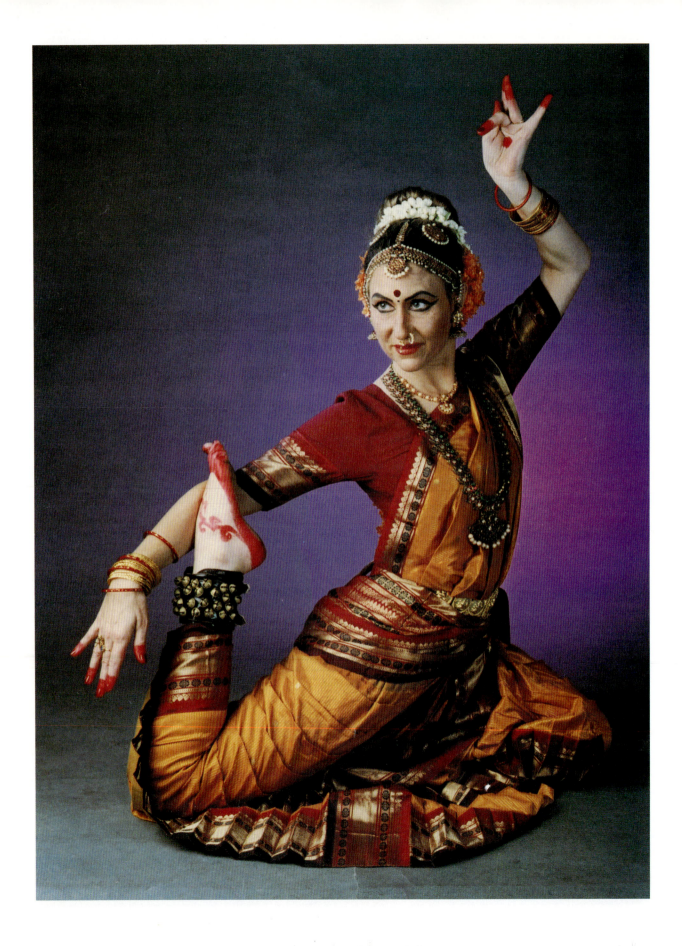

A YOGA
of Indian Classical Dance

A Yoga
of Indian Classical Dance

The Yogini's Mirror

ॐ

Roxanne Kamayani Gupta,
Ph.D.

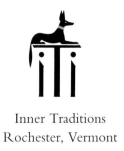

Inner Traditions
Rochester, Vermont

Inner Traditions International
One Park Street
Rochester, Vermont 05767
www.InnerTraditions.com

Copyright © 2000 by Roxanne Poormon Gupta

All rights reserved. No part of this book may be reproduced or utilized in any form or by any means, electronic or mechanical, including photocopying, recording, or by any information storage and retrieval system, without permission in writing from the publisher.

LIBRARY OF CONGRESS CATALOGING-IN-PUBLICATION DATA
Gupta, Roxanne Kamayani.
A yoga of Indian classical dance : the yogini's mirror / Roxanne Kamayani Gupta.
    p.   cm.
ISBN 0-89281-765-8 (alk. paper)
1. Dance—Religious aspects. 2. Dance—India. 3. Yoga. 4. Yoginis—Attitiude and movement. I. Title.
GV1783.5 G87 1999
613.7'046—dc21   99-049252

Printed and bound in Hong Kong

10 9 8 7 6 5 4 3 2 1

All asana photographs and Dance of the Panchabhuta photographs
by Kevin McGowan.
All color dance photographs by B. K. Agarwal.

Text design and layout by Virginia L. Scott
This book was typeset in Bembo with Bauer Bodoni and Cochin as the display typefaces

Contents

Acknowledgments
vii

Preface
ix

INTRODUCTION ❧ Understanding *Yoga* and *Indian Classical Dance*
1

ONE ❧ Discipline and Desire
My Initiation into Indian Spirituality
8

TWO ❧ Dance of the Gurus
Meetings with Remarkable Men and Women
32

THREE ❧ Stillness at the Center
The Yoga of Indian Dance
51

FOUR ❧ The Dance of Yoga
The Sixty-Four Yogini Asanas
59

FIVE ❧ Yoga of the Emotions
Spiritual Dimensions of Indian Drama
150

SIX ❧ The Dance of the Yogini
Tantric Dimensions of Indian Classical Dance
162

SEVEN ❧ Yoga of the Elements
Nature, Culture, and Spirituality
173

Bibliography
190

Dedicated to Ganesh Baba
Om Ganapataye Namah

Acknowledgments

Spanning three continents, many of the people I love have been involved in the creation of this book. Its conception took place a few years ago while I was meditating in front of a photo of my guru, Ganesh Baba, at La Vieux Salidieu Yoga Centre near Lucon, France. I am grateful to my extended guru family there for their continued affection and support.

I completed the bulk of the writing on this book while living with my dance guru, Bala Kondalarao, at Kuchipudi Kalakendra, Vishakapatnam, India. Bala has been a constant source of inspiration for this book and in my life as a whole. In addition, I have been extremely blessed by Guruji, Amma, and the community at Devipuram, and by Sarasvati Devi, a great humanitarian, civic leader, and patron of the arts in Vishakapatnam. Heartfelt thanks also to dance photographer B. K. Agarwal.

My affectionate gratitude goes to photographer and collaborator Kevin McGowan, without whose enthusiasm and patience I might not have carried through on this project. Love to Joseph DeVita and Richard Burger for the generous use of their beautiful garden in Rochester, New York, for the *asana* shootings. The dance of the elements photos were all taken in the Finger Lakes region of upstate New York, my birthplace, a land where my family on both sides settled more than five generations ago, and where the spirits of the Hodonoshonee, "People of the Long House," have played with me since childhood. To my parents and all my ancestors—thank you for my life!

Last but not least, I am indebted to editor Susan Davidson for her patience and skills, and to publisher Ehud Sperling, a true friend and brother in spirit. To my teachers, family, and friends past, present, and future, I offer this book from the heart.

Preface

I couldn't have put it better myself. Daya Krishna, one of India's most distinguished and respected living philosophers, in conversation recently reflected with me upon the nature of intercultural communication. He expressed the view that to reach a true *understanding* between cultures, one had to fall in love. This book, then, is first of all a love story. It is my own story—one that tells how, more than twenty-five years ago, I traveled halfway around the world to become completely immersed in India, submitting myself to its religious and artistic disciplines. But the love story does not end there. This book is an attempt to share some of the important aspects of the highly developed disciplines I encountered, and to offer new theoretical and practical understandings of what Indian culture offers us in the West.

As a scholar of religious studies and anthropology, I am well aware that this book marks a departure from the standards of academic research, for even though it is based on years of study, travel, and field experience, it is also extremely personal and subjective. When at a young age I adopted Indian culture as my own, I cultivated an identity that contrasted sharply with both my American upbringing and my vocation as a student of religious studies. My early university training taught me to keep my experiences and beliefs separate from the subject I was studying, an agenda with which I always struggled. Fortunately, in recent years the feasibility of scholarly "objectivity" has been seriously challenged by new developments in the humanities and social sciences, and so it has become increasingly possible to write in one's own voice, even within the academy.

Nonetheless, I have written this book with a general, rather than a scholarly, audience in mind. As a scholar my thinking and writing focus primarily on establishing distinctions between various terms and categories related to religion and other cultural phenomena. But in this book I am equally interested in understanding the *connections* between the same terms and categories as they are *subjectively experienced*. It is my wish to communicate with a broad audience, especially with those for whom these disciplines may speak on more practical levels.

This book, then, is about more than what I know. It reflects who I am. In choosing to adopt another culture and religion as my own I have had the privilege of immersing myself in many worlds—the mythological world of the East, where I have found my spiritual home, and that of the West, the place in which I was born—as well as their modern and postmodern milieus. Although these worlds overlap, at times they are contradictory and hard to bridge. While I consider myself a convert to Hinduism, I must clarify that the Hinduism I practice, the religion I have inherited from my teachers, is necessarily as mixed up as I am. (This is arguably true of many Hindus born into the culture today, though the blend may be quite different from mine.) The Hinduism I practice is decidedly not Sanatan Dharma (the path of Eternal Truth), nor orthodox in any sense. (In solidarity with the many heterodox movements that have arisen within the tradition, and insofar as I reject fundamentalism of any kind and also recognize that I have not divested myself of my Christian upbringing, I sometimes call myself a Protestant Hindu.) Having been initiated into both kriya and tantra, I adhere to a Hinduism that is more than tolerant; it is highly reflexive: it reflects upon itself rather than taking itself to be the only truth, or even the superior truth (as in Sanatan Dharma). Even as it posits the existence of an underlying nondual reality, the Hinduism I practice recognizes that the world you see is very much determined by the lens through which you see it, and that one's subjectivity is literally and figuratively bound with the nature of the objective world of experience.

Primarily my claim to being a Hindu arises from practice rather than ideas, from the fact that yoga and Indian classical dance are the twin spiritual disciplines that have shaped my life's narrative, the story of a journey that is both collectively shared and idiosyncratically private. For most of my life I have taken my experiences somewhat for granted, but in recent years I have been surprised to discover that many people—those who have attended my dance performances, the students in my yoga classes, and even my academic students—have expressed interest in learning more not only about the disciplines I practice but also about their cultural contexts, how I came to learn them, and what insights I have gained.

While I see myself, in the writing of this book, as a translator of Indian culture, I recognize that my ideas may not necessarily be identical to those of someone born and raised in India. I therefore hope that I have not greatly misrepresented any native points of view in articulating my own. While I cannot imagine what my life would have been without India, I nonetheless hope that this book points beyond my particular experience to the larger transformative possibilities of delving deeply, and respectfully, into the teachings of the planet's oldest civilizations.

INTRODUCTION

Understanding *Yoga* and *Indian Classical Dance*

This book, *A Yoga of Indian Classical Dance: The Yogini's Mirror,* discusses the relationship between two distinct Indian spiritual disciplines. The yogini's mirror is a particularly apt image for what the book endeavors to convey, for the yogini is a powerful female archetype in Indian tantric mythology and thought. A spiritual initiatress, her distinguishing quality is her enchanting dance, which partakes of both creation and transcendence. She dances in both nature and culture, and her dance reflects each back to the other. The yogini's dance is both supremely sexual and sublimely spiritual, manifesting spontaneously within ancient and elaborate structures. Although the yogini is female, she exists in men as well as women; while women seek to embody her energy, men find her the irresistible object of desire. Ultimately, should a man come to possess her, he finds that her dance has also always been his, existing within his own awareness.

One of the most important classical texts on Indian dance is the *Abhinaya Darpana,* or "Mirror of Expression." Written by Nandikeshwara somewhere around the tenth century, this treatise describes various techniques used on the Indian stage. Seeking to adapt some aspects of Indian dance in an entirely new context, my own text mirrors the classical tradition even while departing from its strictly traditional formulations. For finally, a larger, metaphoric sense of *mirror* lies at the heart of this book, a metaphor familiar to both the aesthetic and tantric traditions of India. *Mirror* refers to the process by which we can become more fully aware of our projections in the theater of life, for the self as "performer" not only projects outward to the "audience" but simultaneously reflects inward upon its own nature. The mirror, therefore, represents a coming to consciousness such as that found in tantric yoga practices. In this book I offer the narrative account of my own process—philosophical reflections and practical yogic techniques—hoping that a reader might find in the mirror of another culture some reflection of her or his true nature.

Indian classical dance is one of the oldest dance traditions in the world. More signicantly, it is the oldest *living* dance tradition associated with any of the world's major religions. On the basis of Sanskrit texts that described and systematized the dance in India as early as the second century A.D., we know that the actual practice of sacred dance is much older. Based on archaeological evidence, there is even widespread speculation among Indian scholars that the dance, like yoga itself, has its roots in the ancient culture that predates Hinduism as we know it.

Classical dance in India evolved over the centuries to reflect changing Indian concepts of self and the world. It flourished during the early classical period (fourth to eighth centuries A.D.), when temple and court complexes were at the center of powerful Hindu dynasties, kingdoms designed to reflect and maintain a divine order here on Earth. At that time dance played a central role in people's lives as entertainment, education, and sacred ritual; *devadasis,* women whose lives were dedicated to dance in the temples, enjoyed power and religious prestige within the society. The dance survived under Muslim rule, which established itself in North India by the twelfth century. However, under British colonialism Hindu kingdoms declined, and so began a period of stagnation for Indian dance.

Around the time of Indian independence in 1947, various regional styles of dance were revived and reinterpreted within the context of nationalism, and *classical* took on new significance. As an educated ruling elite sought to define the new national identity, clear-cut determinations distinguished the so-called folk arts from the classical arts of India, especially in the realm of music and dance. Within this hierarchy, one reflecting the aesthetic and cultural values of the western world as much as those of Brahmanic Hinduism, that which is deemed "classical" is by definition considered more sophisticated and developed, conforming to abstract rules, and therefore of higher status.

The notion of "classical" hence introduces certain political dimensions to the world of Indian art. In order to garner India's prestige throughout the world, in the 1940s the dance style of Bharata Natyam was developed from the temple and court dances once performed by devadasis (temple dancers) and court dancers throughout South India. A social movement launched and headquartered in Madras took the art of dance out of the hands of the devadasis. Being stripped of their ritual status, these dancers were suddenly regarded merely as low-caste women, and were condemned as prostitutes by the British. Their positions within the temple were abolished with the willing help of British-educated upper-caste Indians. The art was saved, but also somewhat reinterpreted, by this western-educated upper-caste elite. For these and other reasons, today, especially in South India, the classical dance traditions are largely dominated by male Brahman gurus.

Kuchipudi, the dance style I practice, is named after Kuchelepura, the village of this particular dance's origin in Andhra Pradesh. While Kuchipudi adheres to the standards of the *Natya*

Sastra—the definitive and ancient Sanskrit treatise on dance from which all classical dance traditions in India take their basic form—and boasts an unbroken lineage of hereditary teachers and performers hailing from the village since at least the seventeenth century, it too has been revived and reformed in the past forty years, resulting in some substantial changes to the art form. For hundreds of years, Kuchipudi was a dance drama style limited to Brahman males who dressed and danced as women as a type of spiritual practice. Although it shared many of the same themes and basic styles of movement, Kuchipudi was considered more prestigious than the dance of the devadasis, since it was performed by upper-caste men. Yet following the example of Bharata Natyam, Kuchipudi underwent "reformation" in the early 1950s, and women began performing it for the first time. Although in this generation the Kuchipudi tradition still remains largely under the control of male Brahman gurus, the most important of whom descend from the traditional families of Kuchelepura (now commonly known as Kuchipudi village), there are now a few very accomplished non-Brahman female gurus, my own teacher, Bala Kondalarao, foremost among them, who are leaving their mark on the tradition.

With its introduction into the West through westerners like myself studying in India and Indian dancers beginning to establish dance schools in the West, Indian classical dance now enters the postmodern age, a transition that will undoubtedly result in innovations. This book, an interpretation of the dance as a kind of yoga, represents such a new development; there is no traditional framework in which yoga and dance are combined in this way. This book therefore represents my own creative synthesis of the way the two have come together in my own life, the result of many years of traveling and studying both dance and yoga in India. On a more theoretical level I also present something of a challenge to the mainstream Hindu tradition, using tantric categories to critique the tradition from within, and to hold Indian religion and art to its own self-professed ideals.

In this book, *yoga* refers to a path or discipline leading to spiritual liberation. It is a general term covering several different practical approaches and philosophical schools within India. The term *yoga* is based on the Sanskrit root *yuj,* "to yoke," or "to bring under control." My hatha yoga guru, Apa Pant, used to say that yoga is nothing more or less than yoking the limited individual will to Universal Being. For this reason, yoga is much more than physical exercise. It is a holistic way of relating to the body that involves an increasing awareness on all levels: the physical, the mental or "psychic," and the energetic or "spiritual" dimensions of the human organism. Yoga unites the functions of each of these bodies, as well as their balanced interrelationship under a central organizing principle called Self (what we in the West often refer to as our "higher self").

The supreme spiritual goal of yoga, then, is enlightenment, a state in which one is permanently tuned, or yoked, to the universal will. So while yoga makes it much easier to achieve whatever worldly goals one sets for oneself, the highest spiritual level is concerned not with the fulfillment of desires but with their cessation. True freedom exists not in imposing one's will upon the universe but in finally surrendering one's limited will in favor of the universal.

However, first one must have something to surrender. To withdraw the senses from outer objects and engage the inner world, accessing ever more subtle layers of reality, is the method of yoga. One's experience of the inner world will vary depending upon the type of yoga practiced. For jnana yogis the inner world is accessed through increased mental control and the fine-tuning of one's logical thought processes, a harnessing of the intellect for transcendent insight. In bhakti yoga the concentration is on the invocation of emotion toward a particular deity in order to transform "lower" desires into "higher," or ultimate, human concerns. In kriya yoga specific techniques or mental exercises are used to lead the individual consciousness into mystical states of expanded cosmic identity. Tantric yoga systems do the same, specifically utilizing powerful external tools such as *yantras* (abstract diagrams), *mantras* (sacred sound), and psychosexual imagery as "launching pads" to cosmic consciousness. There is no clear-cut distinction between these different types of yoga; each includes defining elements of the others. The main difference is in where the emphasis is placed. Hatha yoga is usually seen as the most physical type of yoga because of its emphasis on bodily postures, but if one moves deeply into hatha yoga, it too leads to transcendental realms of experience.

On the physical level, hatha yoga develops a total body consciousness that extends inward to various bodily systems: skeletomuscular, respiratory, circulatory, digestive, and even excretory. Yoga *asanas,* or physical postures, combined with breathing, energize the entire organism, promoting health and total well-being through increased circulation. The practice of asanas also results in clarity of mind and increased awareness. Once this awareness develops, heightened bodily sensitivity begins to influence all interactions with one's environment. On the most basic level, once you become aware of the internal physical realm it makes you conscious of what is going into the body—what you are ingesting (food, drink, air, and so forth) as well as what you are (or are not) eliminating. There also develops a natural urge to detoxify. You find that you don't have to force yourself to pay attention to what you are eating or how you are living; your body will automatically begin to reject that which is harmful to you.

With practice this internalization process begins to work on the subtle or psychic body as well, affecting thoughts and feelings. As you become more inner oriented you become aware of the way images, words, and thoughts affect you. By focusing inward you become more conscious of both what you are psychically taking in and what you are putting out. Hence you become more discriminating about your interactions with your environment, the kind of people you closely associate with, the places you go, the activities you engage in, and so on. This is a discrimination based not on external characteristics but on levels of energy. Trusting your intuitions, you begin to feel your resonance—or lack of it—with all that surrounds you. This "intuition" is nothing more (or less) than the development of increasingly subtle levels of perception.

With enough practice, physical postures, the yoga asanas, become a meditation. These postures begin to take on symbolic significance. Many of the traditional asanas of hatha yoga are named after various animals in order for the practitioner to psychically connect with the qualities of being those animals represent.

The postures release the latent energy of these symbols, giving rise to some extraordinary experiences, even to *siddhis* (psychic powers). Any system of yoga that emphasizes siddhis works primarily with the subtle or psychic body. Through the practice of hatha yoga alone you may start to experience so-called extrasensory perceptions, although these are not magic but are instead the logical outcome of heightened conscious awareness. Information in the form of subtle clues begins to register directly in the unconscious and automatically influence your decision-making processes. Premonitions, synchronicities, and even déjà vu occur when the body, mind, and spirit are fully aligned with Universal Being and when there is minimal inner conflict to obstruct events from happening according to one's higher purpose.

But this comes about only through discipline, control of the will. Internalization and increased sensitivity automatically lead to a deepening sense of control over one's physical and mental processes, as well as one's spirituality or "greater self" development. In one sense it seems that, through the discipline of yoga, your life becomes much more controlled, much less free. But this sense of control in no way comes from an external source. It is a kind of renunciation or sloughing off of those things that are no longer necessary to who you are. It is you yourself taking control as your conscious will takes charge of the direction of your life. Through yoga one comes to gradually control one's desires from within, eventually to yoke one's individual will with that of the universal will. According to Indian tradition, it is rare that we can achieve this on our own. It is believed that the universal will therefore manifests itself first and foremost through the guru, or spiritual master.

Guru Brahma Guru Vishnu Guru Devo
  Maheshwara
Guru Saksat Paramguru Tasmai Guruve Namah
(Guru is Brahma, Guru is Vishnu, Guru is Lord
  Siva Maheshwara,
To that Guru, the Highest Manifestation of
  Reality, I bow)

For those who are not ready to assume full responsibility for self-control (and few are), the external guru provides the role model and guide until the time is right for one to realize that the true guru exists within. Yet here a gap between theory and practice can easily arise, because many gurus will counsel their disciples to do one thing while they themselves do another. The student, if he has doubts about the guru, may think him or her a hypocrite, but it may instead be the case that the disciple is at a totally different level of development than the teacher. Nonetheless, devotion is not the equivalent of slavishness. When the inner guru develops to a certain point, the disciple will not hesitate even to go against his external guru's counsel to follow his inner voice. This is all part of the spiritual growth process.

For practical purposes the spiritual body or transcendent realm can best be conceived of as the realm of pure energy. The aim of spiritual or transcendental meditation practices is to attune to that realm on the level of vibrations. Here yoga uses abstract symbols with minimal content to represent energy, since the intent is not mental understanding but direct experience. These abstractions take the visual form of geometric yantras and, more important, are aurally manifest in certain vibratory sounds like *bija* mantras, syllables whose sound qualities are designed to catapult awareness beyond thought.

While for discussion's sake we can separate out the physical, the psychic, and the spiritual objectives and techniques of yoga, in reality there is no such separation: the three levels overlap and interpenetrate one another. Our experience of their disunity is in direct proportion to the extent to which we are all living unbalanced lives. Therefore, whichever aspect an individual chooses to work with has everything to do with one's background (not only in this life but in other lives as well, according to Hindu thought), as well as one's goals and aspirations.

The ego or limited consciousness can easily raise objections and place obstacles in the path to this unity, even for those who are motivated by the highest spiritual goals. For example, the kind of heightened sensitivity that results from yoga practice means more awareness of pain as well as pleasure. When the ego reacts to this possibility from the standpoint of fear, we will tend to opt for less rather than more feeling, and, expecting the worst, begin to harden ourselves. We then build up our ego defenses, some of which can actually mask as ego-inflation—several religious techniques of prayer and meditation that deny body and the feelings have developed within various traditions, all in the name of detachment or some similar notion of transcendence. Even yoga can be misused in this way. Because it involves development of the will, yoga can easily degenerate into an exercise to prove that the will can suppress all feeling in order to obtain a kind of superhuman status. But attempting to attain the status of a god without understanding what it means to be human is a travesty of the Spirit. Denial of emotion in the name of God or any other power only prolongs ignorance and suffering of the self and others.

Becoming more conscious, hence coming to balanced terms with pleasure and pain, is at the heart of what it means to be human, and is essential to the development of both wisdom and compassion. Wisdom involves insight into the nature of your own existence, while compassion relates to understanding where you fit into the whole picture—your relationship with others and the world. The right combination of wisdom and compassion leads to true freedom and bliss as consciousness expands and a variety of options you never dreamed possible open up to you. The expansion of your inner world finds its reflection in the outer world as well.

Nonetheless, many people begin yoga practice and find that they are not ready for the changes that start to occur, precisely because of the increased responsibility that the whole process demands from the individual. Depending upon the circumstances, such an awakening may call for a total change in lifestyle, causing one to grow away from one's friends, family, or current occupation. Unable to make such a radical change, some people leave the path, perhaps to come back to it years later. Only then do they realize that the inner voice had not really gone anywhere. Once awakened, consciousness can be ignored only temporarily; it can never be put to sleep again. It will wait patiently, for whole lifetimes if necessary, for you to come around again and heed its calling. However, in most cases there is no need for drastic transformations. You can pace your degree of involvement in yoga in order to gain its maximum benefits on whatever level you are functioning. It is possible to practice yoga merely for its physical benefits, but if you continue, it will no doubt eventually lead you deeper into the unexplored territory of the Self.

Dance is very much like yoga. It may be argued that this is true of any kind of dance, but in the case of Indian classical dance, this is straightforwardly so. Like yoga, it involves work on the physical, psychic, and spiritual levels, and in fact requires a balancing between these three if it is to succeed in its higher purpose.

In the following chapters I will expand upon the nature and significance of this relationship between yoga and Indian classical dance. I start at the beginning, with my own story. In the first two chapters, "Discipline and Desire" and "Dance of the Gurus," I narrate how I was initiated into the disciplines of dance and yoga, and the manner in which they eventually converged in my life. In chapter 3, "Stillness at the Center," I discuss the relationship between Indian classical dance and yoga both within Indian culture and as subjectively experienced on three levels of being: physical, psychic, and spiritual. Chapter 4, "The Dance of Yoga," introduces the actual physical hatha yoga asanas that I have developed over the past twenty-five years out of my dual practice of dance and yoga.

Chapter 5, "Yoga of the Emotions," discusses the spiritual dimensions of Indian dramatic theory, offering techniques that may be applied to one's daily yoga practice. In chapter 6, "The Dance of the Yogini," I delve further into the tantric dimensions of Indian classical dance, focusing on the relationship between the temple dancer and the yogini in historical and religious terms. Finally, in the last chapter, "Yoga of the Elements," I offer a meditation on the relationship between culture and nature, between body, psyche, and spirit in the natural world, which I hope will lead to an expanded understanding of both yoga and dance.

In Indian goddess-worship rituals, one of the important objects offered to the goddess is a mirror. In this, my personal synthesis of ancient Indian traditions, I make my own offering. I hold up a yoga of Indian classical dance as a mirror to India and to the world, so that we might all come to catch a glimpse of our own divine nature.

ONE

Discipline and Desire
My Initiation into Indian Spirituality

From the beginning India has known the secret of desire: that desire itself lies at the heart of life, of creation, of creativity and manifestation. Without desire the world would cease to exist. But then the Buddha was born in India, and taught that all life is suffering, and that desire lay at the root of all suffering. For without suffering there could be no pleasure, no beauty, no nature. Hindu India, with all her wisdom, could never deny this truth, but neither did she as a civilization ever choose to look it straight in the face. For all her love of the infinite beyond, India's attachment to creation—here and now—has held her in thrall. Out of her great and fertile desire she has given birth to one of the richest cultures this world has ever known. Christopher Columbus discovered America while looking for India. I discovered India while looking for my self.

This is the story of how my desire led me to discipline, how I found what I was searching for in and through my gurus, the teachers who established my practice and shaped the way I see the world. Looking back at my life now, it seems nothing happened by accident, as if everything had been carefully planned in advance.

I can't remember exactly when India first dawned on me. We lived in a small rural community in upstate New York in the days when there was no global studies curriculum, and where no one I ever knew had given a second thought to such a place. Yet I have memories from high school—seeing the Beatles and Mia Farrow on some television talk show with Maharishi Mahesh Yogi, a giggling man with a long white beard, and me fascinated and doubtful, wondering what that was all about. Me, the spring of my senior year, falling half-asleep in a film in sociology class and suddenly jolting awake as I inexplicably *recognized* the image on the screen: a half-naked old man sitting by the side of a river, back straight, eyes closed. I knew this place as if I had been there—not long, long ago but yesterday. I knew that this place was holy, and I could not for the life of me understand why I knew that. These were the sparks, the earliest flickerings of deep memory, the beginnings of desire, and they were soon forgotten until the following year when I was a student at Syracuse University.

I had originally gone to the university to study journalism. It was the early 1970s and, like many of my generation, overnight I found myself critical of everything around me. Suddenly the media seemed little more than a hypocritical game, and my desire to be a journalist waned. Nothing seemed more important than searching for answers to life's ultimate questions. It only took one course in eastern religions during my freshman year for me to decide to major in comparative religious studies. During my sophomore year I studied Hindi and started reading the Bhagavad Gita in my spare time. One day I spotted a poster advertising Indian classical dance; a few nights later, on a snowy evening in January, I attended the recital. The dance was held in Crouse College, performed to some very scratchy recordings of M. S. Subbulakshmi, the most famous of all South Indian carnatic vocalists. What is amazing in retrospect is that the first Indian dance I ever witnessed turned out to be Kuchipudi, the style I would eventually study. The odds were against this coincidence, for in those days Kuchipudi was much less well known than the other major classical styles such as Bharata Natyam, Kathak, or Kathakali.

The music notwithstanding, as soon as the dance began I was transfixed, totally spellbound, entranced. However, as the evening progressed I began to experience a strange anxiety—it dawned on me that I could never be content to simply watch this dance. I wanted very much to try it myself, an idea that to my rational mind seemed preposterous and totally impossible. Here I was, the daughter of working-class parents who, thanks to a scholarship, had been fortunate enough to escape her small town in upstate New York to attend a major university. The pressure of choosing some practical vocation for my life constantly nagged at the back of my mind. And yet suddenly I was filling with this intense desire to—to what? Become an Indian dancer?!

Since in those days I considered myself a devotee of Lord Krishna, halfway through the concert I found myself playing Let's Make a Deal with God. With all sincerity, a prayer formed inside me: "O Krishna, if I could somehow learn this art I would dedicate my dance to your praises forever!"

Walking home that night I could never have dreamed how my life would unfold. For after the initial bright flame of longing burst within my consciousness, perhaps owing to my doubts regarding any possibility of my wish's ever coming true I let go of the idea almost as suddenly as it had arisen.

I now recognize in that moment of desire not only the beginnings of my career in dance but a foreshadowing of my involvement in yoga as well. As an idealistic and intensely searching eighteen-year-old, my spontaneous and completely unselfconscious wish to immerse myself in the dance and to undertake it in a spirit of dedication to deity were some of my earliest steps on a spiritual path. Another essential ingredient was also present. Without knowing it my rational mind had served me well in creating the necessary state of detachment so that the universe could take it from there.

And that seems to be what happened. Events transpired to make my dreams a reality. That spring

I discovered an academic program offered through the University of Wisconsin that would enable me to spend my junior year studying in India. Since I had already studied Hindi for a year at the university, I applied to go to Banaras (Varanasi), the holy city located in North India. I was admitted to the program, but only on the condition that I instead go to South India, to Vishakapatnam, a city on the east coast in Andhra Pradesh. I accepted, albeit with reservations, since this would mean studying a different language. I did not know at the time that that language, Telugu, was the language of Kuchipudi, the dance I so wanted to learn.

I spent the summer in the intensive study of Telugu. Then, a few weeks before we were to leave, we were informed that the program was canceled owing to visa problems. I was crushed. It was at that point that my professor, Velcheru Narayanrao, a native of Andhra, encouraged me to go to India on my own. With his encouragement and the permission of my professors at Syracuse—but much to the chagrin of my parents—I made up my mind to travel alone to Hyderabad to study with Dr. Natraj Ramakrishna, a well-known master who specialized in temple dances of Andhra.

The trip to India was a huge step in my life. I was only nineteen years old and had never traveled outside of America. Wearing a plaid dress and Buster Brown shoes, I boarded the plane in New York; in those days the flight took close to twenty-four hours, with a stop in Beirut. I was already in a state of disbelief; now it seemed as if Air India's 747 was a giant womb delivering me to another world. With only the name and address of a family in Hyderabad, I arrived in Delhi to heat, noise, and confusion in September of 1972.

My plan was to undertake an independent academic study of Indian classical dance in order to write about its cultural and symbolic significance, and only secondarily to undertake practical training. Despite my dream of learning to dance I didn't dare set my sights too high. Although I loved to dance I had no formal training, apart from a year or two of lessons when I was a child. And despite having been a cheerleader in high school, I did not consider myself to be either athletic or particularly coordinated; I had always identified more with my mind than with my body. I went to India thinking I would be satisfied if I could learn some basic movements and a simple dance or two. If not, I thought at least I could develop a little of the grace that seemed to come so naturally to Indian women.

Being a straightforward American, as soon as I arrived in Hyderabad I was anxious to contact the guru, find out how much the fees were going to be, and join the class. But my Indian hosts informed me that this would never do, that I would need to go through certain channels, beginning with a proper introduction. First they would have to send word to request an appointment.

When the appointment was granted, my host "father," Muktevi Lakshminrao, went to speak to the guru and state my purpose, but the guru refused the request to meet me. He said he was not interested in teaching women anymore because every time his female disciples reached a certain age they would get married and discontinue the dance. Later Lakshminrao went again to plead with him, but the guru would not relent. Finally, a few weeks into my stay, just when I was beginning to lose hope, the guru sent word to bring me to the dance school. It seems that while traveling in a car one day he had seen me walking on the road, wiping the sweat from my brow, and had felt sorry for me. Rightly so. Despite all the ways in which I had tried to prepare myself, I was suffering greatly from culture shock and stomachaches. I was sick from the heat, frightened of the cockroaches in the bathroom, and tired of being stared at like some kind of freak. I was homesick and lonely. Still, the idea of going back to America never entered my mind.

When I finally got to meet the dance guru it was an utterly frustrating experience. The entire time we were there the guru spoke only to my Indian "father" and hardly looked at me. I was told that I would attend class every day, morning and evening. I quickly realized there was no question of learning a "little" dance: it was all or nothing. This was my first lesson in understanding the cultural framework of the art—the significance of the guru and the inequality inherent in the guru-student relationship. If one wants to study a traditional Indian art, science, or religion, one has to accept the principle of the guru's superiority. The guru holds the power that comes from possessing the desired knowledge. Submitting oneself to the discipline necessary to obtain that knowledge is the true meaning of the word *disciple,* and is a process that is often hard on the ego.

The traditional nature of Indian culture dictates that the techniques, rules, and guidelines for any discipline are to be maintained as strictly as possible from one generation to the next. Despite the presence of Sanskrit texts and other treatises in regional languages governing various disciplines, Indian traditions were largely transmitted orally because the texts themselves were in the hands of the guru. It was his job to interpret the texts for the student until the student had established his own mastery. The guru is seen as the repository of both theoretical and practical information, as well as transcendent insight. It is for this reason that he is given so much respect. We were instructed to refer to our teacher as "Master Garu," or simply "Master" (*garu* being a Telugu honorific term).

I soon began attending dance class for three hours every morning and another three hours each evening, except on Sunday. The degree to which I saw beauty when watching the dance was the degree to which I felt pain when I first started actually practicing it. How could something that looks so graceful feel so completely awkward and physically unnatural? I was amazed that there were no warm-up exercises; we went into the steps straight off. We danced on sealed concrete floors, stomping our legs with force but attempting to keep the feet relaxed enough to make a slapping sound. The hardest part was getting used to the basic position, which involves turning one's knees fully out to the side and bending the legs. (This was a real killer.)

It seemed that no matter how hard I tried I wasn't getting it. When I concentrated on my leg positions, my hands would relax. Counting the beats, I would forget to smile. I didn't think I would ever be able to move my head from side to side as Master could! Within a few weeks I was completely discouraged, absolutely convinced that I was doing terribly, that I couldn't possibly learn the dance properly. Every day after class I would return to my tiny room, shut the door, and cry miserably.

One day soon after I began my studies, Master called me into his room. I was fully expecting him to tell me that I was wasting my time as well as his and that I should give up my ridiculous attempts. Instead, much to my surprise he demanded to know why I had lied to him, telling him that I had never studied Indian dance before. Stunned, I replied that I never had studied the dance. He said he found this very hard to believe, given the ease with which I was learning. Was I sure I hadn't studied somewhere before? Shocked, I insisted that I had not. Then it struck me, and I began to laugh out loud. It was the cheerleading! In fact, the more I thought about it the more the similarity of some of the movements seemed uncanny. "Cheerleading?" he asked. "What is that?" I had to think about how to explain it. Finally I replied that it is like a kind of dance performed by young girls to a chorus of shouts while boys are playing sports. I even demonstrated a cheer for him. He then asked, "Why do they do this?" I again had to search my mind for an explanation: "To unify the crowd in order to send energy to the team." Later as I thought about our exchange I realized that cheerleading is not all that different from classical Indian dance even in this regard. Indian temple and court dancers also "sent energy" to the "team," namely the deity, the king, and the ruling elite, as a part of temple or court ritual, and were thereby believed to maintain the order of the kingdom. In each case, decorated women not only performed a function but also became symbols of the kingdom they served.

In high school I had been a cheerleader for three years, making the varsity team when I was a sophomore, but I was so small that I felt more like the mascot. When most of my friends on the squad graduated and I was elected student council president my senior year, I quit cheerleading for politics. However, even in later years when fashion dictated that any self-respecting feminist confess and repent her cheerleading past, I never complied. I wasn't built for competitive sports, so I had much preferred shouting and dancing on the sidelines. Ours was a small school, and so cheerleading did not carry the same kind of social weight that it seemed to in other places. I still have no regrets. The exercise and emotional outlet that cheerleading provided not only kept me sane during a turbulent adolescence but also prepared me to study dance halfway around the world.

But for my Indian friends there was another explanation of why I took so easily to Indian dance. Hearing my story they immediately related to it in terms of *samskaras,* the tendencies inherited from a past life. They said that I must have been a devadasi in a previous birth. Otherwise I would never have had such an immediate reaction to the dance performance I saw, nor an opportunity to fulfill my desire to learn it myself. Since I have no way of either proving or disproving their theory I accept it as a kind of personal myth, indicative of my deep connection to Indian culture, for undoubtedly my going to India to study dance was the beginning of a new life for me.

One month into my training Master explained to me that there were certain rituals associated with the art that must be maintained. Serious dance practice commences only after performing *gajja puja,* a ceremony in which the guru ties bells onto the ankles of the student. At this time the dancer offers obeisance to Lord Natraj, the form of Shiva as Lord of the Dance, and to the guru himself, the offerings made in the form of *daksina,* or ritual gifts. The ceremony was to be held only after I had learned a few of the movements from a temple dance called Ganapati Kautam, in honor of Lord Ganesh, the elephant-headed deity known as the remover of obstacles. Ganesh is traditionally invoked at the beginning of any important undertaking.

There was a long list of items for me to furnish for the ceremony. They included *pusupoo* (turmeric), *kumkum* (red sindoor powder), camphor, a coconut, fresh flowers (preferably jasmine, marigolds, and roses), perfume, seven kilos of rice, sweets, a pair of high-quality *dhotis* (the four meters of white cloth worn by Master), and *guru daksina* (money offering). On a day and time chosen for auspiciousness, I arrived at Master's house wearing a new white and pink *saree* and flowers in my hair.

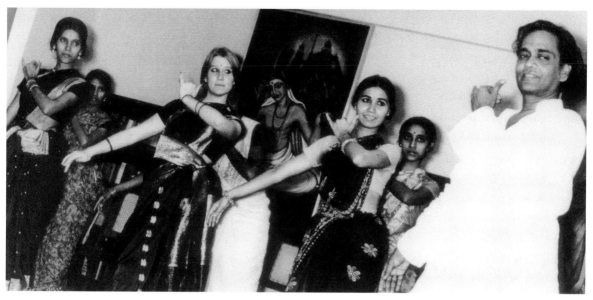

Abhinaya classes at the Sangeet Natak Akademi, Hyderabad, January 1973. Standing in a basic "Krishna" pose (left hand signifying his flute), I keep my eyes on my guru, Sri Natraj Ramakrishna.

The bright yellow turmeric was mixed with water and the thick paste was rubbed on my feet. On top of this the red powder was used to make a *swastik*, an ancient symbol of fertility. The turmeric and kumkum were also used to make a yantra on the dance floor. Over the yantra the rice was piled in a mound. After offering prayers in front of the deity I was made to stand on the rice and, after Master had tied the bells, to symbolically take my first dance steps. (The rice was later distributed to the poor.) Finally I offered the coconut, sweets, flowers, perfume, clothes, and money to Master, and knelt to touch my forehead to his feet. Thus began my official initiation into Indian classical dance.

The classical dance taught by Natraj Ramakrishna is known as Andhra Natyam, the dance performed in and around the temples of Andhra Pradesh since ancient times. This includes the dances of the devadasis, performed before the deities in the temples; Perini Tandavam, a martial dance performed by men in certain Shiva temples to prepare the troops for battle; and Kuchipudi, a dance drama enacting mythological themes, once performed only by men in the temple courtyards. While Kuchipudi was actively being revived and performed by many other artists, especially those from the village of Kuchipudi itself, many of the temple dances were dying out with the last devadasis, since the practice of dedicating women to serve in temples had been outlawed in the 1930s. Perini Tandavam was a dance that had been completely forgotten for hundreds of years. Natraj Ramakrishna reconstructed the dance using old manuscripts and the temple sculptures at Ramappa, an eleventh-century Shiva temple near Warangal. His most famous disciple in the study of this dance was Kelam Sudarshan Rao, who at that time was just a boy of sixteen living in *gurukul* style, cooking for Master and running all his errands. I would sit and watch Master choreograph the Perini Tandavam, asking Sudarshan to try out various movements. Sudarshan became my first close friend in India.

Every morning he would sneak me bread and honey from the kitchen and sometimes steal out of the house to visit me. Some years later I learned the basics of Bharata Natyam from Sudarshan. He became one of my principal informants on the inside world of Indian dance.

Natraj Ramakrishna, who when very young had been a court dancer himself, was especially famous for *abhinaya,* or the art of facial expression. He told me about how his patron, a maharaja near Nagpur, might request him to show any of the nine *rasas,* or archetypal emotional states, at any time. In this way he had developed the ability to laugh, or to cry actual tears, on demand. He also told us about a dance to Ganapati where colored powder would be sprinkled on the floor and the image of an elephant would be created from the dancer's feet. He encouraged me to meditate on the dance carvings on the walls of temples and to understand the connection between dance and visual arts. Reading more about dance I became interested in yoga as well, for a distinguishing characteristic of Indian sculpture is the portrayal of *prana,* or life force. The images in ancient Indian temple sculptures look to be filled with breath, as if the subjects had inhaled and were holding their breath for all eternity.

Several months into my study I met a man who was practicing hatha yoga. He offered to teach me a few asanas and basic breathing exercises. I took him up on his offer but time, and my guru, did not permit me to pursue yoga seriously. Although the attitude is now changing in urban areas, most Indians view yoga as something mainly associated with *sadhus* (holy men) and renunciates and hence not appropriate for ordinary people, especially women. Whenever I would talk about yoga Natraj Ramakrishna would insist that dance itself is a yoga, that one could attain siddhi (extraordinary powers) and even *samadhi,* the final state of total

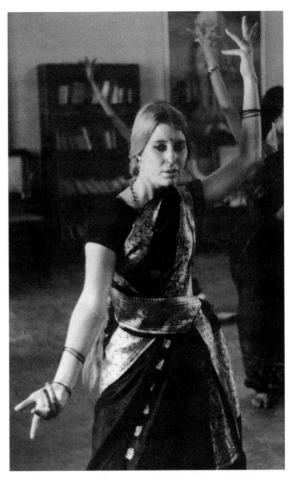

In dance class, 1973. I am wearing my new green silk Banarsi saree, a "souvenir" of my first trip to Varanasi, the city most sacred to Hindus. Even during the earliest stages of my training I tried to attune myself to the spiritual dimensions of the art and used dance as a means for inner development.

absorption and nonduality, through dance. He told me of such an experience he had once had—while dancing he felt his consciousness leave his body and float in the air. He could see himself dancing from above. Through total absorption in dance he had overcome the duality between the actor and the witness, the performer and the audience.

I took Master's words seriously, and so began to delve into various aspects of Indian spirituality in order to understand the deeper meaning of dance.

Sometimes I would take a vow of silence for a set number of days in order to deepen my concentration and powers of observation. Even though I would warn everyone around me in advance, it would still drive them all quite frantic, and they wondered if I was losing my mind. In India a wide variety of religious practices are tolerated, but only within appropriate contexts. To see their visiting American student take so earnestly to devotional practices meant for holy men or devout widows was simply too much for most of the families that were looking after me. Another time I decided to live only on consecrated food, *prasad,* the food offered to the gods at temples and then returned to devotees as leftovers: hardly enough to live on, let alone dance on. That was the final proof to some that I had gone off the deep end, for in India there is no greater social sin than to refuse food that is offered to you.

Immersed in these kinds of trials I let my imagination soar freely, and new ideas would come to me spontaneously, the validity of which I would be immediately convinced. For example, one day during a lengthy bus ride it simply dawned on me that music and dance have the power to heal. I later informed my guru that if a dancer were absolutely pure in spirit and intent and offered her dance to the gods, it should be possible for her to cure everyone in the audience of all disease. When I look back on those days now I realize how impossibly naive I must have appeared when I would go running to Master with these revelations. But on the other hand, I cannot say that I was so far from the truth. Today the healing potential of music is beginning to be taken seriously even in the medical field, and given a new anthropological emphasis in the field of religious studies, an appreciation of the shamanic role of dance in healing is beginning to emerge.

The Devadasi

As a research scholar as well as a dancer, Natraj Ramakrishna had worked hard to gain recognition for the old and forgotten artists of the state, especially the devadasis who lost their status and patronage when temple dancing was outlawed. The British saw the devadasis as little more than prostitutes. While the colonial rulers had no problem with prostitution, maintaining large brothels on the outskirts of their own settlements, their Christian sensibilities were offended at the notion of women being dedicated, literally married, to the deities of Hindu temples. Their lack of comprehension of an art form that combined eroticism and spirituality led them, in conjunction with "modern" Indian reformers, to outlaw the institution of temple dancing in the early part of this century.

However, there were some South Indian lovers of the art who saw the danger in censoring the dance along with the dancer. Some of these were western-educated Brahmans, the upper-caste intelligentsia of the colonial period. Equally influential were the Theosophists, a spiritual community originally founded in the late nineteenth century by the Russian-born mystic Madame Helena Blavatsky and later presided over by the English freethinker and Indian freedom fighter Annie Besant. The Theosophists were a mixed community of Europeans, Americans, Australians, and Indians whose world headquarters were centered in Adyar, Madras, the same place from which the major revival of Indian classical dance would take place around the time of Indian independence. Rukmini Arundale, an urban-educated, high-caste Indian woman who at an early age married George Arundale, one of the leading officers in the

Theosophical Society, was undoubtedly the most influential figure of the dance revival movement. At a time when Indian dance was looked down upon by the British and many Indians, she had the nerve to clean up the art, so to speak, and perform it in a respectable and sophisticated venue. In this way the dance came out of the "closet" of the temples and into the limelight of the modern stage. The Russian prima ballerina Anna Pavlova was influential in this development: the story goes that Rukmini Devi approached Pavlova for ballet lessons, and the great ballerina encouraged Rukmini to learn the dances of her own culture instead.

At the time, some version of Indian dance was already known in the West through the vaudeville stage and other orientalist theater productions playing throughout America and Europe. As early as 1909 Ruth St. Denis, one of the leading figures in the founding of American modern dance, was performing her own rendition of Indian dance. Known as Nautch, the dance was a bastardized form of Kathak that had been taken from the courts of North Indian rulers into the parlors of the British raj. Nonetheless, the fact that such public figures as Pavlova and St. Denis (and later St. Denis's husband, Ted Shawn) praised the art provided the kind of official—that is, western—recognition necessary for Indians to reconsider the value of their own traditions. At the time of Indian independence Rukmini Arundale founded Kalakshetra, a traditional dance school in Madras from which many of the leading figures in Bharata Natyam (a name she coined) later emerged. At the same time at least a few of the traditional performers of the art—most notably the famous Bala Sarasvati, who was born into the devadasi community—were able to continue performing and teaching, even though the institution of temple dancing had been officially abolished. During this movement toward its revaluing, the spiritual nature of Indian dance was highly emphasized as its selling point, countering its tainted reputation associated with temple prostitution. Eventually other dance styles, such as Kathakali and Manipuri, Odissi and Kuchipudi, were designated as classical. The government soon began to support the revival of these arts. However, most of the traditional performers of the art were left behind. My guru, Natraj Ramakrishna, had spent a great deal of his youth learning dance from the devadasis of his small town in coastal Andhra Pradesh. After achieving some success in his career as a scholar and performer of dance, it became his lifelong project to give something back to his devadasi teachers. Through his untiring efforts, the remaining elderly devadasis of the state were eventually granted modest government pensions and, in some cases, recognition for their artistic achievements. As part of this larger project, I was fortunate that during my period of study with him Natraj Ramakrishna arranged a special three-month seminar on abhinaya (facial expression) featuring Srimati A. Buli Venkataratnama, a devadasi from East Godavari district.

Venkataratnama was in her early sixties when she came to us, but she was still an imposing figure—tall, straight, and very beautiful and dignified. She walked like a queen. She wore traditional silk sarees, and as is the custom among wealthy women of the region, several chains of gold, coral, and pearls on her neck and clusters of diamonds on both sides of her nose. She also wore a *mangala sutra,* the traditional marriage thread, with two *talis* or round gold medallions indicating her married status. For as a devadasi she was *sumangali,* the eternally married woman, incapable of becoming a widow, since she was married to Vishnu, the god of the temple to whom she was dedicated as a young girl. Accordingly, she also had two tattoos branded on her upper arms reflecting her devadasi status—on the left the outline of a conch shell, and on the right a wheel, the two sacred signs of Lord Vishnu, the Preserver of the Universe. The palms of her hands and the bottoms of her feet were stained orange with henna; her kohl-blackened eyes sparkled with mischief and revealed a formidable and proud nature. Despite her years Venkataratnama was still dancing and, through her art of facial expression, could transform herself into a young girl. I remember once during a public lecture-demonstration she was sitting cross-legged on the dais, enacting through facial and hand gestures a song in which a *nayika* (heroine) was pleading for her lover Lord Krishna to come to her. Venkataratnama as the heroine was so convincing that in the middle of the song a man from the back actually thought she was calling him, and he got up and started for the stage! The audience laughed as his face flushed in embarassment.

When teaching, Venkataratnama used to ask us to sit on the floor opposite her and imitate her expressions. By using only her eyes and facial muscles she would convey many emotions—shyness, desire, indignation, sorrow, jealousy, and wonder, changing from one to another with ease. Later we would practice these within the context of a song, such as a traditional *padam,* in which a heroine was chiding her lover for his neglect or expressing jealousy over another woman. Through this great teacher I came to appreciate the depth that comes with experience, and her example helped me to consider aging in a very different light. For in spite of her age Venkataratnama was the very embodiment of sensuality and spirituality, passion and wisdom, like a living goddess.

I soon became attached to Venkataratnama and

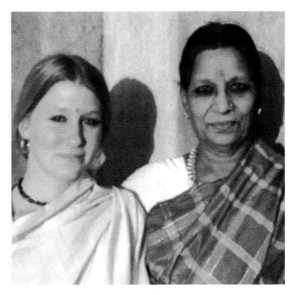

I imitated my teacher the devadasi Venkataratnama in every way. I wore kajal on my eyes, chewed paan, and tied my saree like hers. But while she wore gold, pearls, and diamonds, I could only afford glass beads. Here our photo is taken outside my little room, which she was kind enough to grace with her presence. In India it is considered a great honor if a teacher visits a student's home, and accepts from the student even a cup of tea.

began to follow her around like a shadow. Every day after lunch I would go to her room and take *paan,* a tender green betel leaf spread with white lime paste and folded around a small piece of betel nut. Chewed slowly and kept in the mouth, paan turns the tongue, teeth, and lips a bright red color. Taking paan is a common habit in North India, but in the south it is more of an occasional indulgence. As it is believed to be a mild aphrodisiac, it is considered romantic for a woman and a man to offer paan to each other after dinner. In one of the most famous dances of the Kuchipudi repertoire, the Krishna Sabdam "Swami Ra, Ra" (Lord, Please Come to Me), the heroine tempts Krishna with paan, but he won't take it until she places it in his mouth herself. Venkataratnama kept a solid silver box in which she stored all the ingredients for her after-meal ritual. Her teeth were permanently stained with paan juice, adding to her courtesan persona. To be like her I too used to chew paan and have red teeth, something my fellow students considered quite rustic and decadent.

Venkataratnama proudly followed many such traditional customs. They were a part of who she was. For example, before eating she used to set aside a tiny portion of her food as an offering to her Lord and "husband," Vishnu. That way whatever she was eating became prasad, sacred leftovers such as those given in all temples in India. Some of Venkataratnama's customs challenged my western way of seeing the world and opened my eyes to the radically different ways that various cultures react to typical human situations. In our class there was a student who had come from another state. She was in her early twenties and very high-strung, the life of the party at one moment and depressed and withdrawn the next. One afternoon she entered class and fell down on the floor in a fit of possession, staring off into space with a terrified look on her face, unblinking and totally immobile. After a few moments she broke out into a hysterical crying fit. Venkataratnama entered, took one look at her, and seemed to know what to do. She and another devadasi took the girl away with them to their room, where I later heard that they administered some kind of an exorcism that included hitting her on the joints with a bamboo pole. I was shocked. I went to my guru and told him, "This girl needs help, not a beating. She needs a psychiatrist!" He said "This is India, not America. We don't have such doctors here." To my surprise, after the indigenous treatment the student returned to her familiar self and didn't seem to resent the devadasis for what they had done. Today she is a well-known dance teacher in a neighboring state. Of course in the many years since this experience my thinking about traditional healing methods has greatly expanded, though I believe I would still find such rough treatment hard to accept. However, it seemed to have worked.

What was most satisfying about my relationship with Venkataratnama was that it transcended the limitations of spoken language. She spoke no English, and my Telugu was most inadequate to broach the ideas I wanted to discuss with her. Therefore our communication was conducted almost entirely through body language. I will never forget one episode in which Venkataratnama brilliantly conveyed her point without speaking a word. I used to have a crush on my guru but, since he was more than twenty years my senior, I felt that he never took me seriously. One day he said something dismissive that hurt my feelings and I came running into Venkataratnama's room practically in tears. Simply by holding up her thumb, she gestured, "What's wrong?" Pouting, I replied in my broken Telugu, "He treats me like I am a little girl!" Her eyes flashed. With her mouth full of betel, she lifted her left elbow and, with her right hand, reached over and jiggled the sagging flesh that hung from her upper arm. She raised her eyebrows and gestured with her eyes for me to take a good look at it. Then her face took on an expression that said so much about growing old—pathos, regret, and resignation—as if to say, "Count yourself lucky, young lady. Wait till you have this." It was so dramatic I could not help but burst out laughing at her, and at my own foolishness.

While Venkataratnama was given respect as a teacher, most of the students felt a bit uncomfortable around her. This was probably due to the social stigma attached to devadasis. I was well aware of the devadasis' reputations as prostitutes, but I knew there was much more to it than that. One day I played innocent and asked Venkataratnama where her husband was. Surprisingly she

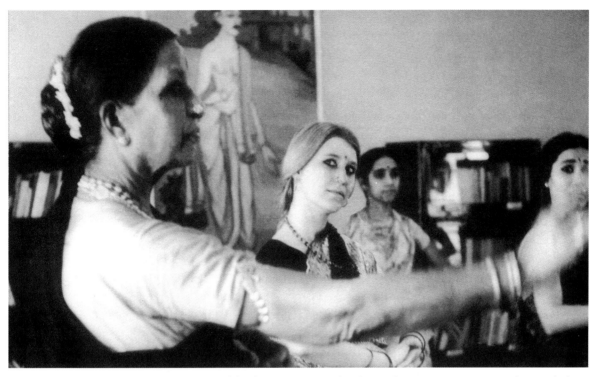

At abhinaya classes we learned the subtle art of facial expression. Here devadasi Venkataratnama instructs us in how to get the attention of the hero by calling him to her with an intimate wave of her hand. Although she was over sixty years old at the time, she carried herself like a young queen.

didn't say, "He is at home in the temple," but rather she laughed and with a grand gesture stated, "He has gone to the Himalayas." Perhaps she was referring to her wealthy patron rather than her god. Soon afterward I got up the nerve to ask my guru whether what people said about the sexual freedom of devadasis was true. He told me that while devadasis were married to the god of the temple, they were free to go with other men. It was very common for a devadasi to be "kept" by one man who supported her like a second wife. Others had several patrons from the educated elite of the community. According to Master, from some men devadasis took money, to others they gave it away. It all depended on "their wish," he said. He stressed to me that devadasis were highly educated women, well-versed in classical Telugu and Sanskrit, in Hindu *dharma* (religion), and in the "sixty-four arts," such as painting, cooking, poetry, decoration, and so on. Not long ago pilgrims to temples used to roll in the dirt that devadasis had danced on in order to absorb some of their *shakti*, or powerful sacred energy.

But not all devadasis were created equal. Some were little better than servants in the temple whose duty it was to fan the idol or walk in front of the deity when the image was taken out in procession for special holidays. Others, like Venkataratnama, who were particularly intelligent, beautiful, or talented, would perform dance in front of the sanctum of the main deity. Such a devadasi could become quite famous and wealthy and she would in turn make generous grants for temple construction and development. Devadasis who served in the temples could also become court dancers if they gained the ruler's favor. By custom the local ruler, whose laws the temple complex reinforced and supported and who would in many cases be treated as a living representation of the god himself, would have rights to the "first night," or consummation, of the young devadasi's marriage to the deity. Since their sexuality was for ritual and not procreative purposes, devadasis developed their own methods of contraception. One was the insertion of a betel nut into the uterus, the prototype of the IUD.

In short, devadasis were neither helpless victims nor harlots. Indeed, it may be argued that they were the most educated and "liberated" women of medieval India. South Indian legends abound with stories about devadasis, some of whom reached prominent positions in various kingdoms. It was only when temple patronage declined and the devadasis were forced into a monied economy that their status suffered and they became anachronisms, forced to find other ways to support themselves.

My time with Venkataratnama soon came to an end. Upon the completion of our seminar the students gave a performance, and for the first time I danced in public. Venkataratnama was excited at the prospect of dressing me. On the morning of the program she took me into the bathroom and gave me a ritual bath. With her own hands she washed my hair with *kunkaitikai,* or soap nuts, known in North India and in the West as *shikakai.* Then she rubbed pusupoo (turmeric) on my limbs and rinsed it off with water. On holy days women in Andhra Pradesh bathe with turmeric, which lends a slight tint to their brown skin. Bright yellow is the most auspicious of all colors, being associated with Lakshmi, the goddess of fertility and wealth, but turmeric's traditional value in the culture may also be related to its antiseptic qualities.

With my white skin, after my bath I looked like a walking marigold. Luckily the stage makeup masked it.

After the program it came time for Venkataratnama to return to her village. Sudarshan and I tearfully accompanied her to the station. At that time she invited me to come with her to her village, to see her large estate (lands given by her wealthy patron, a *zamindar,* or "landlord of the village"), her house near the river, her only daughter and granddaughter. She promised me that if I came, she would teach me songs from the Gola Kalapam, a Kuchipudi drama based on the dialogue between a Brahman and a milkmaid. But Master refused permission. As much as he had done for the devadasis, he could not rise above the societal prejudice toward them. He told me, "We never go and stay in the homes of devadasis. It wouldn't look nice." I could have taken Venkataratnama's invitation anyway, but I didn't want to go against my guru's word. To this day I regret the lost opportunity, for Venkataratnama died a few years later and I never saw her again, except in my dreams.

After Venkataratnama left, the hot season set in. It was during this period that my life took a turn that I could never have predicted. It was a time of transformation during which I had profound insights into the spiritual dimensions of Indian dance, and into life itself. I have spent half a lifetime trying to reconcile those revelations, mystical experiences that were later dismissed, or at least radically tempered, by my graduate studies in religion and anthropology. My education severely challenged my innocent enthusiasm for unbounded spiritual experience. But before I had ever heard the word *orientalism,* before any professor had enlightened me to the fact that I had lost all objectivity by committing the cardinal sin of "going native," I unwittingly wandered into psychic regions inhabited only by fools and saints, where the difference between the two no longer matters.

The Long and Winding Road

For the longest time I thought I didn't need a spiritual guru, since I had dance as my path. However, at a certain point I began to question this assumption. It started with an interest in Sai Baba, whose picture I began noticing everywhere. Indeed, his photos are displayed in homes throughout India—especially in Andhra Pradesh, which is his home state—but heretofore I had paid no attention to them. Soon I began taking his repeated appearance as a sign. I began praying to Sai Baba, asking him to reveal himself to me if he was my guru. I even drew a huge *mandala* with chalk outside the door of my rooftop apartment as a "landing pad" on which for him to psychically arrive. One day he was due to visit his temple in Hyderabad, so I vowed to meet him there and have his *darshan,* a meeting of spiritual exchange. I got delayed, and by the time I reached the temple the gathering was already breaking up. As the huge crowd was exiting, I was entering, against the stream. At the gate an austere woman in a white saree asked me where I was going. I told her I had to meet Sai Baba. She said he had already left and that I too would have to leave now. "That's impossible," I said. "I know I am going to see him today." I stood in the yard near the temple and resolutely vowed not to move from the spot until I saw Sai Baba. About ten minutes went by. There were still so many people leaving it took all the will I could muster to stand my ground. After several moments of enduring disapproving glares from the woman in white who had insisted he had gone, I abruptly turned my back to her. Much to my astonishment there stood Sai Baba right in front of me, not three feet away, looking straight at me. I jumped, then quickly took a *rudraksha mala* (sacred bead necklace) from around my neck and offered it to him. I looked into his eyes and mentally asked, "Are you my guru?" He held the mala for a moment and then handed it back to me. As he looked at me the word *no* immediately came from within my own mind. The answer was clear and unequivocal.

Since then I have had very little interest in Sai Baba, yet to this day I wonder about my meeting with him. Was it really Sai Baba? He is well known for having the siddhi (power) to appear in several places at once. If what I saw was some kind of apparition I am truly impressed, because he stood before me as clear as day and even took the mala from my hands. And if it was him, why didn't any of the other people who were moving about notice him or try to approach him? Why did we seem to somehow be alone? Whatever it was, after having the darshan of Sai Baba my life began to get very interesting.

A phenomenon common to many religious traditions has to do with sickness and suffering. Mystical experience and/or religious conversion is often the result of a life-threatening condition, after which the self seems to reconstitute itself in a new configuration. So it happened with me. Within a month of meeting Sai Baba, the scorching heat of summer set in and I developed a fever. It began low and imperceptible and soon began to rage. It eventually topped off at a temperature of 105 degrees Fahrenheit (which was still considerably less than the temperature outside). In retrospect I realize I had developed all the symptoms of typhus, a disease that comes from eating contaminated food. It is true that I had not been very careful about my diet. Although I was a strict vegetarian and so did not eat any meat, I prided myself on my ability to eat the hottest pickles, and I ignored the less than hygienic conditions of some of my friends' kitchens. In my sickness I couldn't keep anything down, and eventually began to vomit even after I drank only a few mouthfuls of water. Although I became severely dehydrated and delirious, my doctor (at whose ineptitude I now marvel) could do nothing except give me injections of vitamin B. He said he could admit me to the hospital, but I would probably be worse off for it. After a week of taking my temperature every few hours, my motherly landlady, Lakshmi, became so alarmed that she went to Master and pleaded with him to do something, but it seems he just sat there looking worried. Furious, she told him that if I died it would be his fault for doing nothing.

It wasn't that Master didn't care; he just didn't know what to do. I was the one who didn't much care that I was wasting away. Although I was burning up inside, the delirium gave me a kind of ethereal feeling, the almost pleasant sensation that I was connected to my body by only a thin thread. A part of me was watching the whole drama, curious to see how far I could push the outer boundaries of consciousness, and where it would lead me. One night I was lying on the balcony under the stars, trying to sleep in the heat. Gazing up into the night sky, I saw everything begin to turn, slowly at first, then faster, and then faster still. The spinning stars formed themselves into a tunnel, an inverted funnel pulling me upward into its center. It was a hypnotic feeling, not at all unpleasant, but suddenly something in me resisted and it struck me what was happening—how very easy it would be to simply let myself go, to let my soul be sucked out of my body. With great difficulty I got up and went inside to find Lakshmi. I knew her energy would keep me grounded.

I eventually reached the limit of my suffering. In a few weeks' time I had grown so weak I could no longer walk without help and had lost so much weight that I looked like a stick. Finally the decisive moment arrived. It came in a dream early one morning.

I was walking down the street in Hyderabad. A beggar woman, old and bent, was slowly approaching from the opposite direction. As our paths were about to cross, she looked up at me and I casually glanced at her face. Suddenly she took on a very ugly and threatening demeanor. As I watched in horror and fascination, she began to grow into a dark and towering figure, sprouting hundreds of heads and mouths, protruding teeth and tongues, breasts and legs, her many arms bearing weapons of destruction. I felt panic grip me in the pit of my stomach, and instantly knew that I had no time to waste. In a split second it came to me that no matter how frightened I felt inside I should not show it, for she would only feed off my weakness. If I were doomed, at least I would go down with dignity. Struggling to control my reactions, I locked my eyes into hers. Without moving we stared at each other for an excruciatingly long time. Then the words formed in my mind: "As black as she is, that is how white I must become." My eyes still locked with hers, I felt a tremendous power rise from deep within me. Using every ounce of remaining strength, in that eerily slow and dampened dream state I willed myself to grow into a form equal to hers, sprouting heads, arms, and legs, but without weapons, smiling with confidence, free from anger. I felt my feigned fearlessness transform into a deep and abiding calm that radiated outward like a searing light, countering her terror with compassion, becoming the perfect opposite, the perfect complement, the perfect white reflection of her: Her Royal Blackness, my nemesis, my mirror, my shadow. We reached an understanding—it was a crystal moment of true balance and identity. It was the turning point. Standing perfectly still, I didn't blink as I watched her shrink in size and return to the form of an old beggar woman who hobbled on past me. My power slowly withdrew back into the center of my body.

At that moment I awoke. I lay perfectly still as I emerged from the dream, the entire sequence flooding my consciousness in a matter of seconds. I could still hear the distinctive sound that accompanied the dream, one in which no words were exchanged. The sound not only vibrated inside my head; it permeated my entire body. It was the sound of a thousand winds rushing from all directions of eight-dimensional space, harmonized into a single vibration. There is no description in language that can begin to capture its absolute fullness. In later research I came upon the term *anahad sabd,* the "unstruck sound," a term used by the medieval *sants* (saints) of North India to describe the sacred inner sound experienced in advanced meditative states. But I remember it as the sound of the sun, for as I awakened the first rays of the rising sun were shining in my eyes, and I was bathed in sweat: my fever had broken. Amazingly, I was filled with energy, as if I had never been sick. I jumped up and ran downstairs, dreadfully scaring my landlady, who soon ordered me back to bed rest.

A few days later a young couple who lived some distance away invited me to stay in their flat while I regained my strength. Since they had an air cooler in their bedroom, they thought it would be good for me to rest there a few days. The first afternoon in their flat there came a knock at the door and my host's brother said someone was there to see me. "How can that be?" I asked. "Nobody knows I'm here." He replied that an elderly *sanyasin,* a holy man, had come to the door inquiring whether there was some foreigner staying here. He told me that, if I wanted, he would send the man away. By then I was curious, so I went to the verandah to meet the caller. He was an old man in sadhu dress, wearing spectacles and sporting a long white beard. Obviously an educated man, he spoke excellent English. He introduced himself and said that he was conducting research on the relationship between yoga and classical Indian dance. "That's amazing!" I said. "Because I'm here studying classical dance and I am very interested in this subject. How did you know I was here?" He said that the neighbors had told him about me. But this didn't make sense because my friends had only very recently moved into this particular apartment and they hadn't had time to get to know their neighbors yet, so how would they even know I was there?

Our conversation commenced, with him conducting what seemed like an interview. The first question the old man asked was, "What is your impression of Sai Baba?" In light of my recent experience it seemed strange that he would ask about this. I started to wonder whether I had entered the twilight zone. I answered him by saying that I had had Sai Baba's darshan six weeks previous and that, although I was impressed with his miracles, I also knew that he was not the guru for me. He then asked me what kind of guru I was looking for. I replied that I wasn't really looking for a guru, that if my true guru really existed he would find me sooner or later. Staring intently, he went on to ask me a series of questions regarding my spiritual beliefs, which I answered one by one. I felt like I was sitting in some kind of oral exam or admission interview. We spent at least two and a half hours together, but apart from some general statements on spirituality he didn't have much to say about dance. We mostly talked about yoga. Still, I felt very happy to spend the time in *satsang* (spiritual communion) with this holy man, and I gave him a money offering before he left.

The next day I received a letter from some American friends asking me to meet them in Banaras, after which we would all go to the mountains together to get some relief from the heat. I left immediately. It was during this trip to the holy city of Banaras that my life took its most dramatic turn. No sooner did I arrive than I happened to meet a young and handsome Indian man with whom I immediately became intrigued. Although he hailed from a family of prominent scholars, he had left his family to live the life of a sadhu in Banaras. We stayed up all night talking about his guru, an amazing man who had recently left for the foothills of the Himalayas. As we talked I saw my future unfold before my eyes—I knew that he was talking about *my* guru. The next day we went to the Durga temple and exchanged garlands in marriage, and a few days later registered our marriage in the court. My husband then took me to Nainital, where we searched for the apartment where the guru was staying.

After three days of searching I finally met him. He was living in a small apartment above a sweet shop, surrounded by books and handwritten manuscripts, a small man in orange dress, wire-rimmed spectacles, and a long white beard. Having just recovered from a bout with illness, he was being tended by two foreign disciples, a German and an Australian. My guru's name was Sri Mahant Swami Ganeshanand Saraswati, but he was better known as Ganesh Baba. Born of a Bengali father and a Nepali mother, he had been educated at Calcutta University and spoke sophisticated British English through snuff-laden whiskers. Having taken *sanyas*, or final renunciation of his former identity, under the famous Swami Sivananda at Rishikesh sometime in his late thirties, Ganesh Baba was given the title of "Saraswati" by his guru, a designation reserved for highly educated renunciates that indicated his status as an intellectual in the orthodox Dasnami order of Shaivite ascetics. He later attained the parallel title of "Giri" and the status of Mahant, or administrative head, at Alaknath Naga Sanyasi Akhara, Bareilly. As sadhus, Nagas are recognized as fierce warriors rather than intellectuals. Ganesh Baba was both. In his *sadhana* (spiritual practice), he was even more. For he was also a kriya yogi in the Lahiri lineage with a propensity for psychedelics and quantum physics.

As soon as I laid eyes on Ganesh Baba I began to weep. The overwhelming emotion I experienced was great relief, the sense that somehow I had accomplished a very difficult task, had overcome all obstacles in my way, had passed all the tests and was now home free. Baba looked so familiar to me, as if I had known him forever. For one thing, he looked suspiciously like the old sadhu who had unexpectedly showed up at my door just the week before—in fact, the first words out of his mouth were, "Where have you been, my child? I was expecting you for the past few months. I thought I was going to have to come looking for you." This was followed by an outburst of knowing and outrageous laughter, as if he had read my mind. He also looked very much like Mr. Natural, an R. Crumb comic character of which I had been extremely fond a few years earlier. What a long, strange journey it had been to reach him, and an even longer, stranger trip was about to commence! Little did I know then that I had found not only my guru but my animus, the perfect reflection of my ideal masculine self: my beloved grandfather, professor, psychoanalyst, physician, alchemist, master wizard, trickster, and guardian protector.

Baba took his name from Ganesh, the elephant-headed god who is the first deity to be invoked in any Hindu temple or ceremony. Originally a tribal totemic figure, Ganesh was taken up by later traditions as a guardian deity protecting the territory of the main god, be that Shiva, Vishnu, or Shakti. As such, Ganesh is the only major Hindu god who transcends all sectarian differences; mythologically he is depicted as the son of Shiva and Parvati, the original couple. Ganesh combines the fierce strength of an elephant with the wisdom of the highest sage. He is also playful, one of his most popular manifestations being that of dancing Ganesh, and is extremely fond of eating sweets.

Ganesh Baba embodied all these characteristics and more. He saw his role as that of a synthesizer in the Hegelian sense: the creative resolver of thesis and antithesis. Just as the deity Ganesh mediated the differences between various Hindu sects, Ganesh Baba sought to synthesize the differences between all opposites: East and West, male and female, high and low, good and evil. Never one to see the world in black and white terms, and never allowing himself to be categorized, he stood for an infinitely creative approach in which one would be capable of adapting to any circumstance, accepting each moment on its own terms and being open, flexible, able to move with the flow. That was the dance of Ganesh Baba, and the dance of yoga that I too began to learn just by being around him.

I was very lucky to have Ganesh Baba as my *diksha* guru. According to kriya yoga the guru who gives diksha, or "initiation," is of supreme impor-

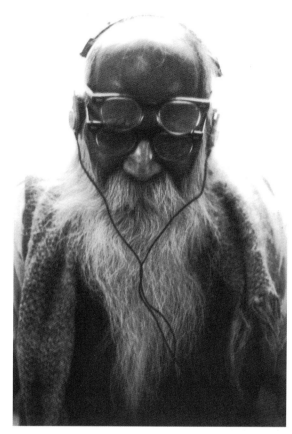

My initiatory guru, Ganesh Baba. As he stood for the creative synthesis of science and religion, he was never one to reject the advances of modern technology. Here he simultaneously listens to headphones while wearing two pairs of "spectacles," one for reading and one for distance. Photograph by Ira Cohen.

tance because he or she administers the jolt of subtle electrical energy that jump-starts the process of spiritualization. The experience of diksha is as if someone had reached into the inner self and turned on the light. Internalization is a central concept in all of the yogic paths. Some conceptualization of inner psychic processes is the starting point from which one can begin to reflect upon one's own consciousness and gain a degree of mastery over one's actions. Only after this is done should one even begin to think in terms of transcendence.

As a member of the Ganeshian crowd I was in good, if somewhat unorthodox, company. At the time they found him most of Ganesh Baba's followers were looking for a one-way ticket out of reality as they knew it. The vast majority were hippies or other similarly disillusioned westerners who had come to India to escape the meaninglessness of their own societies, each with their own story to tell. In the sixties seekers of every kind came in droves to India from all over Europe, America, and Australia. The frontline troops in the international tourist invasion of India, they frequented places such as Goa, Kathmandu, Banaras (Varanasi), Brindaban, Pushkar, and Poona, and made their impact on the local culture as they sought out gurus, sadhus, and other holy men and women—anyone who they thought could offer them "enlightenment." It is interesting to me that the term *enlightenment* also refers to the period in which Europe achieved her greatest glories—the rise of rationalism, individualism, and science that promised progress to the entire globe and in the name of which the conquering of other, "unenlightened" (hence "dark"), territories, such as India and Africa, took place. By the mid–twentieth century, European-style enlightenment fully played itself out in the blinding flash of science's apocalyptic achievement, the atom bomb. Growing up in the shadow of the bomb, disillusioned with the ideals espoused but not practiced by their own governments and religions, many young people ran for cover to the same "primitive" lands colonized by their ancestors, still looking for enlightenment. Except this time they were told that it was to be found, one way or another, within the self.

In the coming years, both during my time with Ganesh Baba in India and nearly ten years after I met him, when I brought him to America, Ganesh Baba shaped my character in ways I could never have dreamed of. I have never talked as much, nor listened as intently, to any human being as I did to him. Sometimes we would stay up all night, me taking notes throughout his soliloquies. Combining scientific and spiritual approaches, Ganesh Baba would teach me from his perspectives on western and eastern philosophy, history, sociology, international politics, comparative religion, Jungian psychoanalysis, physiology, tantra, numerology, astrology, ayurveda, physics, and psychic phenomena. The profundity of his insights would be matched only by his acerbic wit and totally outrageous sense of humor. Never wanting to be considered a goody goody guru, he could curse like any *naga,* or lecture sublimely in an Oxford English accent. With his words he could send his disciples off into the cosmos, or he could make us laugh so hard that we rolled on the ground.

A great defender of "my children, the hippies," he used to say that if it weren't for their protests, the Vietnam War would have continued and would have totally destroyed any moral standing left for the United States in the eyes of the world. He considered marijuana and psychedelic drugs to have had positive effects on western culture, for they helped young people to see through the alcoholic pipe dreams of the warmonger industrialists. Yet he also made many of his disciples stop smoking and using drugs altogether and counseled against addictions of any kind. He warned that without yoga, marijuana use could be detrimental to one's health, and would make the user paranoid. Whereas Timothy Leary instructed an entire generation to "turn on, tune in, and drop out," Ganesh Baba's message was somewhat different. Even though Baba was himself a sanyasin, a renunciate who had left family and home to fully pursue the religious path, he never counseled his disciples

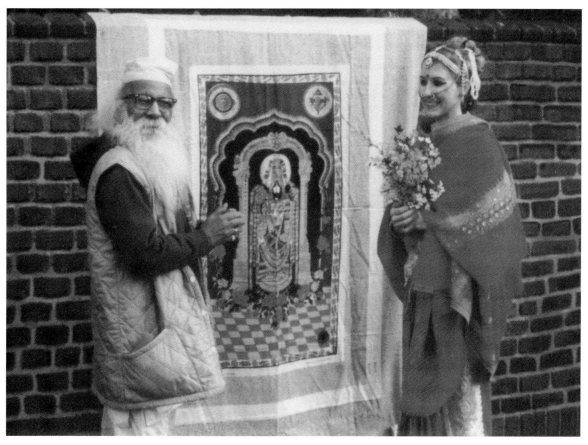

I take Ganesh Baba's blessings before an outdoor performance of my one-woman dance drama, "Madhavi, Courtesan of Puhar," at Houghton House Gardens, Hobart and William Smith Colleges, Geneva, N.Y. May, 1980.

to leave their worldly responsibilities in order to pursue the inner world, or spiritual life. Instead, to those who were running from the West his advice was to use yoga to find oneself, then go home and transform the world.

Kriya yoga, the practice of techniques for expanding conscious awareness, combined with karma yoga, pursuing one's work as a spiritual undertaking and remaining detached from the fruits of that work, were the principal paths Ganesh Baba emphasized, but he also considered some kind of hatha yoga to be important for maintaining what he referred to as the "body-mind machine." Under Ganesh Baba's guidance I began to meditate regularly and to practice hatha yoga more seriously as an integral part of a more holistic lifestyle. He taught me certain positions and exercises, but more important, Ganesh Baba literally taught me how to breathe. "Straight back and proper breathing" were the first lessons in his "higher" education program, known as "the four Ps": posture and *pranayama* (proper breathing) are the basic foundation on which *pronov* (repetition of the mantra), and *pinealization* (internalized visualization) are built. Indeed, these are the bare bones basics of all yoga.

Baba greatly encouraged my practice of Indian classical dance, but being the supreme synthesizer, he urged me to take an innovative approach, not to let myself become totally confined by Indian tradition. He suggested that I combine my dance with hatha yoga, an idea I did not take seriously for many years. To consciously try to do so seemed somewhat forced at the time, though over the years it happened quite naturally, resulting in my own yoga. For the discovery of my true sadhana, I have to give credit to my *adi* (original) guru, Ganesh Baba, who planted the seeds that could take root and grow only after many seasons of watering, through the actual practice of both disciplines.

After marriage and my fateful meeting with my spiritual guru, I returned to Hyderabad alone to complete my dance training. The news of my marriage created quite a stir in the Hyderabad community in which I lived, as did all my talk about Banaras, gurus, and yoga, but nothing could touch the state of grace in which I was living. The blessings just kept flowing. It was at this time that I met my spiritual mother.

Her name was Sarojini Devi. She was a Brahman, the sister-in-law to my landlady. It turned out that she lived practically next door to Sai Baba's temple in Hyderabad, the place where I had had his darshan. But hers was a different path. Every Friday she performed Devi *puja,* worship of the Mother Goddess in the form of Durga. It was a long, elaborate ceremony involving the chanting of the *lalitha sahashranam,* the thousand Sanskrit names of the goddess, while offering kumkum, flowers, incense, camphor, milk, rice, and special food preparations. Every Friday nine women would show up at her house, often complete strangers who had heard about her, and she would treat them with honor, like living goddesses. After she completed the puja the Divine Mother would enter her body, as if in a kind of possession. First Sarojini Devi would begin to yawn repeatedly; then she would start snapping her fingers around her head and, with eyes closed, she would start to weave from side to side. In that state Sarojini Devi would give blessings, healing messages, and predictions. As the goddess she would hold me in her arms like a child, or I would lay my head on her lap because I would start to feel dizzy and weak from the amount of energy passing through me.

We quickly became very close. To her, none of my experiences seemed strange. She told me her own story—how the goddess had come to her in her dreams during a long and serious illness in which she was not expected to survive, how the goddess had saved her, claiming Sarojini Devi as one of her own and giving her instructions on how to worship. The dreams never stopped. She would tell me the latest ones in which she would be distributing huge mounds of kumkum to thousands of people. She felt a tremendous responsibility to heal the world. One day she confided to me that she had lost many children to miscarriages, including a daughter born late in November of 1952, around the time of my birthday. Trying to explain the closeness we felt, she had a theory that I had been originally born to her but then died and immediately went and inhabited the body of my birth mother's child, which was born two months premature. The fact that my birth mother had lost a baby born similarly premature a year and a half before I was, as well as my own six-week separation from her immediately after my birth, led to a distance between us that had never been satisfactorily bridged. From a psychological perspective there is no doubt in my mind that this longing for connection with the mother led me to "Mother" India.

Of course my birth mother did not appreciate Sarojini Devi's version of my genesis, even though my mother would be the first to admit that she has

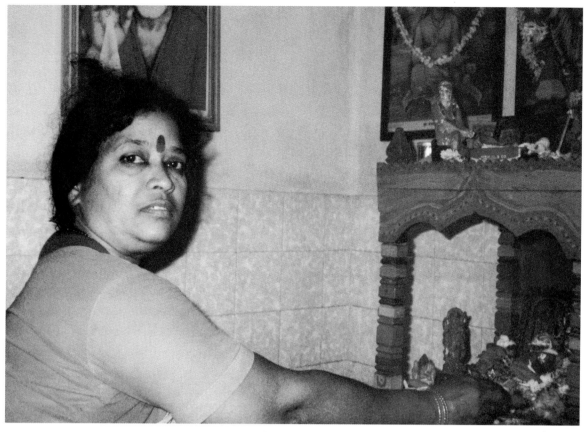

Sarojini Devi, a Brahman woman, at her home shrine, Hyderabad, 1976. A devotee of the goddess in the form of Durga, Sarojini Ma used to perform puja (worship ceremony) every Friday. A variety of women from the city would attend the ritual, after which the goddess would "possess" Sarojini Ma in order to give blessings and advice to those assembled.

always had a difficult time understanding either where I was coming from or where I was going. The two women could not be more opposite, even physically. Sarojini was the archetypal mother, voluptuously full-figured, with long black hair and a face resembling the picture of Durga herself. My mother, like me, was always slim and fair, a somewhat glamorous, coiffed type despite having given birth to six children. She never overate, nor overfed us. In contrast, Sarojini, like all good Indian mothers, saw her kitchen as an extension of her puja room. An excellent cook, she took particular joy in preparing several vegetarian dishes to offer on Fridays, including the goddess's favorite dish—rice pudding made with brown sugar and cardamom. In India food is an integral part of spirituality and is itself worshiped as a manifestation of the goddess. The pride I now take in my own cooking, the pleasure I take in feeding people, and many of the customs I follow are traceable to Sarojini's influence, even though it was my birth mother who so thoroughly trained me not only in cooking but in all the basic homemaking skills when I was young. While in subsequent years I came to address many Indian women as "Amma," or "Ma," Sarojini will always be my first mother in the spiritual sense because it was through her that I was exposed to Devi worship, a devotional practice that would later become my primary religious focus.

By now nearly a year had passed and it was almost time for me to return to America. Master insisted that before I leave I should give my *arangetram,* my first full solo dance performance—a rite of passage for all classical Indian dancers. It was held at Ravindra Bharathi auditorium in Hyderabad, the main performing arts center in the state capital. The newspapers interviewed me and printed my photo, so there was standing room only the night of the program. The performance, two hours long, was a big success. It was the beginning of many programs that I would give in the coming years in America, Europe, and India. Since that first performance I have danced in auditoriums, theaters, lofts, and on makeshift outdoor stages. I have performed for a thousand people in the Government Arts Center in Ljubliana, Slovenia, and for a handful of Quakers in Pennsylvania. I have danced in museums, colleges, churches, and temples. My greatest honors were to perform at the *prana pratistha* (deity installation) ceremonies of two temples—the Sri Venkateshwara temple in Pittsburg and the Sri Rajarajeshwari temple in Devipuram, Andhra Pradesh, South India, as well as at a special ceremony honoring the guru Mother Meera during one of her rare visits to America.

I have never thought of my dance in terms of a career. As much as I love the dance, or perhaps because I love it, I never wanted to depend on it as a main source of income. Of course, as a westerner it would have been difficult at any rate, but other western women have managed to make Indian dance their full-time occupation, and a few have become quite successful. But I have never heavily identified with my role as an Indian dancer. Even though I enjoy performing in public, I have wanted to avoid the highly competitive and politics-ridden world of professional dance. I see dance first and foremost as a sadhana, a spiritual practice. Though it might seem selfish, it is still something I do primarily for myself. I am never happier than when I am in my studio alone, practicing dance, with no one watching except my gods and gurus.

I mention gurus in the plural for, while everyone knows there are countless Indian gods and goddesses, most people have only one guru. But

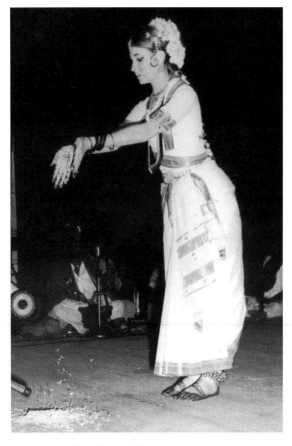

Pushpanjali, the offering of flowers to the stage—the opening dance of my arrangetram (first dance performance) at Ravindra Bharathi Performing Arts Center, 1993. Wearing a traditional nine-yard saree and bells tied on my feet by my guru, Natraj Ramakrishna, I offer prayers to the stage, the audience, gods, and gurus. Photograph by G. Krishna.

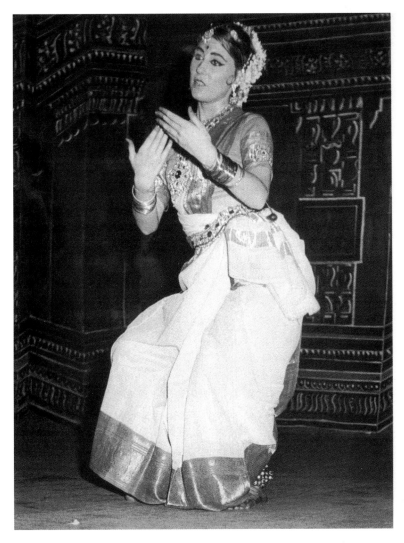

The heroine of a padam, *a devotional poem set to music, beckons her lover Lord Krishna to return to her after a long absence. The dancer uses four kinds of expression to convey her message: words and music, body language, ornamentation, and innate emotions that show on her face.*

thanks to the blessings of my adi (original) guru, Baba Ganesh, I have been blessed with gurus galore. After my initiation into kriya yoga by Ganesh Baba I had the opportunity to explore many kinds of yoga through a series of extraordinary spiritual encounters. Although today most of my gurus are no longer "alive" in the conventional use of the term, I still speak of them in the present tense, for I find that they continue to guide and teach me, and grant me the fulfillment of all my legitimate desires. Although they no longer exist on the physical plane, they exist within me as particular individuated energies, as practical knowledge and a sense of my own higher self.

TWO

Dance of the Gurus

Meetings with Remarkable Men and Women

While some people, even in polytheistic India, swear unwavering loyalty to one god or one guru, I have never been mono- anything. Ganesh Baba used to have a good time making fun of gurus who forbid their disciples to visit other holy men or teachers. Just as he himself had many spiritual teachers, he wanted his students to "feel free." That meant to continue exploring; to have the darshan of as many great souls as possible; to engage in satsang with the disciples of many gurus; to learn to see through the facade of appearances to the inner workings of everything around us. And so I was blessed like Dattatreya Swami, who, according to legend, had twenty-four *upa* gurus, including the wind, the earth, the fire, the crow, the wasp, and the harlot. The message of this traditional story is that if one has the right attitude one can learn from nearly everything in the universe. Therefore no one need suffer for want of a guru, for as it is said, "When the disciple is ready, the guru will appear," even if the guru does not always appear in the form one expects.

These days the very concept of the guru seems to have become somewhat suspect—this is as true of urban India as of the West. It is very much in fashion in America to disavow one's former guru(s) in the name of finding the guru within. But for me there is no contradiction between the guru within and the guru without. Thirty years after the major guru invasion of America many seekers have become disillusioned with the people they have called "Guru" because the latter have failed to live up to the disciple's expectations, moral or otherwise. But I see even those experiences, shattering and painful as they can be, as lessons in and of themselves, part of the spiritual process. It is a mistake for anyone to enter into a relationship with someone they call "Guru" and then proceed to impose his (or her) standards upon the other. This is like playing with fire; but this is a very dangerous game in which the disciple can only lose, because it is only the guru (if he is indeed a guru at all) who knows the rules of the game to begin with. Therefore it is the guru, not the disciple, who gets to break them as well. Of course, this means that the relationship between guru and disciple is *by definition* unequal; it is completely antidemocratic, something that especially goes against the American grain, and yet Americans are the biggest "guru chasers" in the world. This is perhaps because, of all the peoples in the world, we have the least idea of what the larger "game" is all about, despite our religions and rationalist beliefs. On some level we know that we *don't* know.

To enter into relationship with a guru is to enter into a vast and unknown territory, trusting that person as your only guide. There is no guarantee that the territory will be all sweetness and light, as part of the guru's job is to bring you face-to-face with your own shadow, both individual and collective, those unresolved regions of the self that hold us back from inherent human freedom. Yet those of us with Christian backgrounds have a tendency to project only the image of the lily white superego onto our gurus and then wonder why we are so rudely awakened. What may appear to one disciple as betrayal could just as well be a hard but necessary lesson for someone at a different level of understanding. This is not to justify any and all behavior on the part of so-called spiritual teachers, but is only to say that such relationships are hard to judge in black and white terms. As well, the presence of some unscrupulous gurus does not mean that the very concept of the guru must be called into question.

Nonetheless, without understanding the possible pitfalls people are usually in a hurry to give up their power to another human being, perhaps to bolster their egos (their limited selves) by identifying with a force larger than themselves, or perhaps unconsciously believing that they can escape responsibility for their own lives. There is nothing within Indian tradition that says one should surrender without fully understanding who or what one is surrendering to. The Bhagavad Gita, perhaps the most widely read of all Hindu texts, is the story of a great battle, a metaphor for the battle for mastery over one's self. In the story, Krishna, the Supreme Lord, counsels Arjuna, the archetypal warrior, to go into battle putting his full faith in Krishna, but Arjuna is not able to do so until Krishna reveals his infinite Viswa Swaroop form to him. When one bows down in front of a guru one is paying homage not to that person's limited personality, as attractive as he or she might seem, but to the larger tradition he or she embodies, and to the transcendent Ultimate, which is one's own self as well. It is actually the relationship, the process itself, that teaches us who we really are.

The relationship between guru and disciple is extremely intense precisely because it forces you to consciously face a central human question—the whole issue of involvement and detachment, which also characterizes all other human relationships. The unique way in which this is played out between any two individuals is a karmic affair, impossible to judge from the outside (and sometimes even from the standpoint of one who is experiencing it). Many of the things that Ganesh Baba said or did only made sense to me years later. Furthermore, it is not necessary that one should cling to the guru forever. The guru, like the boat, is there to help you cross the river. Once you reach the other shore, you can leave the boat. If the guru

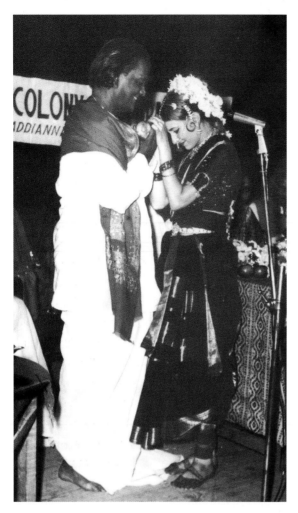

I take my guru's blessings after a dance program in which he bestowed upon me the title "Natya Kala Kaumudi" (Moonlight of Indian Dance). Hyderabad, 1978. Photograph by G. Krishna.

I have been extremely fortunate in my life that each of the persons I have considered as a guru has been an exceptional human being, in addition to being exactly the teacher I needed at the time. Despite various challenges, none has ever belied my trust. They have all displayed an appropriate balance between involvement and detachment. Love tempered with compassion gives rise to wisdom: it knows what is to be gained by letting go, and also knows that, in reality, there is no such thing as separation. There is nowhere we can go to escape who we really are.

The Dance of Jnana, the Path of Knowledge

The path of jnana yoga is one of the easiest paths in which one can get lost. The mind is so endlessly fascinating that it can readily consume all of one's attentions and energies, and convince itself of its own superiority. From the lofty heights of jnana, the ruling elites of the world's greatest religions have constructed complex structures and edifices which have shone with such brilliance that they have sometimes threatened to blind their creators.

For years I had an ongoing but affectionate debate with my late professor and mentor Dr. Agehananda Bharati, in which I questioned the superiority of philosophical systems and orthodox formulations over direct and spontaneous religious experience. Swami, as many of us students called him, was an extraordinary man and a true *jnani* in every sense of the word. Born to an Austrian aristocratic family in the 1930s, he became the first westerner ever to be initiated as a monk in the highly respected Sankaracharya Dasnami order of India. A towering figure—he stood well over six feet tall—he is best known in western scholarly cir-

is really worthy of the title, he or she will be detached and therefore never object to your growing away. Of course, honoring the guru is another matter. As Indians always say, nothing brings worse luck than to bad-mouth one's guru. Sometimes nothing less than complete disillusionment in another human being will remind you of the fact that ultimately your spiritual growth is in your own hands—and if this happens, all the more reason to honor the guru who taught you that lesson.

cles as an authority of south Asia and a pioneer in the field of tantric studies, while in India he is still remembered as an outspoken holy man, the author of a controversial autobiography, *The Oche Robe*.

Born Leopold Fischer, he became fluent in several Indian and European languages while still an adolescent. He was drafted into the German army during World War II. After the war he fled to India, where he first joined the Ramakrishna order, a Hindu renaissance movement headquartered in Calcutta, though this order soon disappointed him with its reformist agenda. After leaving the order he traveled to Banaras, where he took initiation into sanyas (final renunciation) in the highly orthodox Dasnami order. Given the title and status of a learned monk, he earned the highest degrees at Sanskrit University in Banaras, studied music, and went on to teach philosophy at various prestigious universities in south and southeast Asia before returning to the West in the early sixties. He taught first at the University of Washington in Seattle, and finally for many more years at Syracuse University, where he headed the department of anthropology. In his new American incarnation, Agehananda Bharati was a man of many interests, both sacred and profane. A patron of the arts as well as the social sciences, he was brilliant and unorthodox, imposing and outspoken. Without abandoning his spiritual practices, he never tried to hide his worldly preferences—for heated debates, good food, and the company of beautiful, intelligent women.

Although I had met him once before leaving for India for the first time, I really became Swami's student after my return from India in 1973. I suppose that, given his own past, he felt an affinity with me for the culture shock I was experiencing. When most of my other professors thought that I had gone slightly mad, my friendship with Swami deepened.

Yet in the beginning I found the breadth and width of his intelligence quite intimidating. Just listening to him, fascinating as he was, could make me feel small and ignorant. Swami had no patience for what he called "woolly" thinkers. When he found me speaking in generalities he would challenge me to sharpen my critical thinking skills. Once, early on in our relationship, he humiliated me in public by ridiculing something I had said, and that too in a very loud voice. I clearly remember how shaken I was and how I wondered whether I should simply avoid him in the future. Immediately a voice inside me told me that to do so would be simply to go on coddling the ego; that I should instead steel myself for the duration if that is what it would take to learn from this intellectual giant. In later years I realized that the harshness of his words were the way in which he separated the wheat from the chaff, so to speak, and kept his close interactions outside the classroom to a minimum. Because if you were a member of his inner circle, there was no end to his generosity. And even though he was a passionate defender of his ideas, he was never too proud to later change his mind or viewpoint and admit that he had been mistaken.

Swami was not only the advisor for my doctoral dissertation; he was my beloved confidant, teacher, and patron, even during the years I was not part of the university. He was an example to me not only in his life—the courage with which he synthesized his western upbringing with his involvement in Indian culture, and the skills and integrity he brought to his scholarship—but in the way he exited this world as well, for that was the proof of his full stature as a jnana yogi.

With a full teaching load, many academic writing projects in process, and plans to begin the final volume of his autobiography, Swami was suddenly diagnosed with an advanced case of brain cancer in

January of 1991. From the moment he was informed that it was likely he had no more than six months to live, he totally abandoned all academic work. His interest in discussing intellectual topics ceased from that moment on. He immediately retreated into his sadhana and began preparing himself for his final departure.

This was the greatest lesson he ever taught me, a lesson about the priorities of life, a lesson about letting go. While it was largely owing to his influence that I continued in the university to complete my Ph.D., it was also finally his example that has enabled me to maintain a healthy detachment from the world of "publish or perish." As committed and totally involved as I am with my teaching and research, even in my dance, thanks to him I never forget to put it all into a larger perspective. After all, very few published more than Agehananda Bharati, and he still perished. Yet he not only left behind his writings, but for those who knew him well, he left behind a tremendous spiritual legacy as well.

The Dance of Karma Yoga, the Path of Action

It was also through the university that I met the man who I consider to be my true hatha yoga guru—the late Sri Apa Pant, son of the Maharaja of Oundh, the man who developed Surya Namaskar, or the "Salute to the Sun," as it is currently practiced throughout the world. Inspired by Vedic sun-worship rituals that involve a series of mantras accompanied by prostrations, Apa Pant's father, Sri Balwant Rai Pant, created an exercise incorporating hatha yogic elements that would fully benefit the body as well as the mind.

Apa Pant not only taught me the correct way to perform Surya Namaskar and other asanas of hatha yoga; he also taught me the true meaning of karma yoga, the yoga of action. A close disciple of Mahatma Gandhi, Apa Pant was a freedom fighter. A philosopher by nature and a mystic at heart, he served for over forty years as a career diplomat for the Indian government. As the chief Indian officer in Sikkim in the mid 1950s, he was instrumental in obtaining refugee status for the Dalai Lama and the Tibetan community in India, thus influencing the course of history and the spread of Tibetan Buddhism throughout the world. In keeping with his Gandhian vision of world peace, Apa Pant pioneered ecumenism and communication between leaders of various religions. He studied the world's major religions in their original context, meeting with Islamics in Egypt, Roman Catholics in Rome, Tibetan Buddhists, and Hindus of every persuasion, all of which he documented in his autobiographical writings.

I met Apa Pant when he was in his early seventies. He had come to give a talk at Syracuse University, where I was working as Outreach Coordinator, and I invited him to stay at my home. On the way to the car following his talk, I offered to carry his overnight bag. With all the charm that comes naturally to an international diplomat, he said, "Madame, I can not only carry this bag. I can carry you along with it if you like." From that moment on I was totally infatuated.

Our first evening together he regaled my husband and son and me with tales of Tibet, and of Gandhi and Nehru, all of which revealed not only spiritual insight but a passionate love of life. At dawn the next morning Apa Sahib and I did yoga together, and he showed me the correct way to perform Surya Namaskar, along with the accompanying mantras. In subsequent sessions in the following years he refined my practice of other yoga asanas and various breathing exercises, and gave me invaluable insights into the philosophy of yoga, Gandhian nonviolence, politics, and the cosmos in general. After he was awarded an honorary doctorate from Syracuse University in 1989, we toured Maharastra together with a small group of family and friends, videotaping Surya Namaskar as it is practiced in state schools and colleges. On this unforgettable journey I was able to interview various yoga practitioners, including Apa Pant's lifelong friend master yogi B. K. S. Iyengar. In Apa Pant's hometown in Oundh I was honored to receive the blessings of his family's goddess, Ambabai, in their family's private temple, and to perform dance in the museum of fine arts that houses his father's extensive collection of rare traditional and contemporary Indian paintings.

Apa Pant died a few years later. The last letter I received from him, shortly before his death, was filled with accounts of mystic visions and ecstatic experiences as he neared the "ocean of bliss." He considered the letting-go process a thrilling experience, something he had prepared himself for his entire life, and wrote that there was no need at all for me to reply to his letter as he was already in the state where he felt no separation from anyone or anything. As was to happen to me more than once in my life, when he left his body I felt in my guru's passing an immediate shower of blessings in the form of insights, lucky events, and deepened meditation states, and, ever since, I feel an abiding reassurance and presence whenever I choose to "tune in."

The Dance of Aghor Sadhana, the Fearless Path

Whenever I have been deprived of the physical presence of one guru, events have transpired to bring me into contact with another important teacher. It was thus that I met Avadhut Bhagwan Ram, one of the most fully realized human beings I have ever known.

It all began when I was undertaking a graduate research project on *aghoris,* the most radical and heterodox of all Hindu ascetics. Known as tantrics who worship powerful forms of the goddess in terrifying cremation-ground rituals, in India aghoris are a source of great fear and fascination. Since my earliest visits to Banaras I had been interested to find out more about the Kina Rami aghoris, a sect whose headquarters were near my husband's residence. Years later when Avadhut Bhagwan Ram, the sect's charismatic leader recognized throughout India as an *aghoreshwara* (one who had attained the state of liberation through this unorthodox path), came to New York for a kidney transplant, I sought permission to interview him for my research project. What was intriguing to me was how he had given up all radical practices in the latter part of his life and had become a social reformer, a moral force in North India on behalf of outcastes, lepers, women—all those who have been traditionally excluded from both spiritual and material benefits within orthodox Hinduism. As I have always sought to ground my own social and political activism in a spiritual framework, this greatly appealed to me.

I went to interview the guru in the apartment where he was staying, a block from the United Nations, and met him again briefly in his ashram in Banaras the next summer. By then I was so fascinated with him and the larger implications of this radical path that I decided to write my doctoral dissertation on the sect that he headed.

The following November my beloved guru Ganesh Baba left his body, an event for which I was not prepared. By then Avadhut Bhagwan Ram was back in America, and in his presence I cried like a lost child over my guru's death. The few calm words of reassurance the Avadhut spoke to me on that occasion touched me deeply. I became quietly convinced that Ganesh Baba had not abandoned me or my "higher education," but had left me in the care of this guru. Over the next six years, until his own death from kidney-related complications in 1993, I delved deeply into the world of Avadhut Bhagwan Ram and the mystery of aghor sadhana. By the time he left his pain-ravaged body I had achieved a new acceptance of death as transformation, and could fully appreciate the Avadhut's way of putting it: "Gurus don't die. They just go behind the curtain."

My relationship with the Avadhut was unlike that with any other guru. By the time I met him he was in his early fifties and, due to the painful process he was undergoing of burning off the collective karma of his followers, most aspects of his individual personality had been transcended in favor of the countenance of a *boddhisattva,* a Buddha who renounces final liberation until all other souls are similarly enlightened. Perhaps his having the power of the impersonal realm of compassion is why his human interactions with us would shower us with bliss and insight. During the eighteen months I was living near him in Banaras, undertaking research on his sect, I was graced with many experiences and insights. Although he rarely spoke directly to me, whatever questions I had would automatically get answered: doors would open and people would "coincidentally" appear in my life to help me find out whatever I wanted to know. Such occurrences went well beyond my academic concerns. Whatever was happening on the intellectual front was just the tip of the iceberg compared with the changes that were happening within me.

The most extraordinary event took place on my birthday in 1989. The night before, I was walking alone to my room overlooking the Ganges. It was late at night, the moon shining overhead. As I looked down at the peaceful *ghats,* the many stairs leading down to the river, I was struck once again by the timeless nature of the holy city. In a pensive mood, I thought of all the great saints, sadhus, and other holy men and women who had walked on this well-worn path, including my beloved departed guru, Ganesh Baba. No sooner had I thought of him than I was overcome with sadness and longing. I missed him so much! I thought of an episode in *Autobiography of a Yogi* in which Paramahansa Yogananda longed for his guru, Sri Yukteshwar, after his death, and how subsequently Sri Yukteshwar had appeared to Yogananda like the risen Christ. Wistfully I addressed Ganesh Baba in my mind. "Tomorrow is my birthday. If I could have anything I wanted, it would be to spend just a few hours with you, Baba. I would give anything just to talk to you one more time." I liked the idea so much that as I fell asleep that night I indulged myself in the fantasy of sitting and talking with him on the riverbank. "Why not?" I thought. "Anything is possible."

The next morning I was unexpectedly invited out to breakfast by another foreigner staying in our house. She took me to an expensive hotel on the other side of town. Since we had traveled so far, I decided to visit an address near there that had been given to me by someone in the Avadhut's ashram; I had been interviewing one of the Avadhut's disciples when he told me that I should definitely meet his father, a householder who had taken renunciation in his old age. He said that his father knew a great deal about aghor sadhana and other aspects of spirituality. So with notebook in hand, I arrived unannounced. I was invited inside by the daughter-in-law of the house, a woman about my own age who told me in Hindi that she would tell her father-in-law (and guru) that I had come.

When after a few minutes he called me into the room, I was immediately taken aback. There before my eyes was a short man with long white hair and a beard, dressed in the orange dress of a sanyasi and wearing wire-rimmed spectacles. He was the spitting image of Ganesh Baba! I sat down, stunned. Instead of my interviewing him, he began to lecture me, taking charge of the conversation exactly like Baba used to do. The first words out of the old man's mouth—in perfect English, of course—were "What is a guru?" And for the next few hours he proceeded to talk about the concept of guru. In another typical Ganesh Baba gesture, he took out a paper and pen and drew diagrams to illustrate some of his points. I was unable to take notes. Instead, I concentrated intently on the message I knew my guru was sending me from beyond the grave.

One of the metaphors the old man used was that of a clay oil lamp. When the lamp breaks and the fire temporarily goes out, it doesn't mean that fire is gone from the earth. The guru is the flame, not the lamp. The guru is the same flame that burns in every lamp, for all individual fires partake of the universal nature of fire. With the same surety I felt the night I cried in front of the Avadhut, I realized that Baba was now assuring me that he would never abandon me, that he could hear my prayers and would come through for me whenever I needed him. Through the old man he was also reminding me that I should find him now in the Avadhut, because on a certain level there was really no difference between them. Another way of interpreting the episode was that it was the Avadhut himself who, out of compassion, granted my desire to see my guru in something very close to the form to which I was so attached, but in so doing was also reminding me to look beyond the form to the principle.

Caught between these two explanations, I realized that both—or neither—might be "true." They were, in the end, only limited conceptualizations that could never capture the full experience of what had happened. What really mattered was that my dream had come true, my heart's desire was being realized. As I surrendered to the miracle of it all, my eyes filled with tears that then streamed down my face. The old man didn't seem surprised when I told him why I was crying. He inquired about Ganesh Baba's *sampradaya* (lineage), and it turned out that they had met many years earlier at Sivananda's ashram in the Himalayas.

When it came time for me to go, there was no talk of our meeting again. There was no need. With a heart full of love I touched his feet before I left and never looked back.

I can never forget that this event took place during the time that I was under the Avadhut's care in Banaras. While undertaking research on his sect I had heard so many stories of the miraculous events that took place around him, and had other chances myself to witness them firsthand. But it was not primarily the supernatural or miraculous that drew me to Avadhut Bhagwan Ram, nor is it that which commands my eternal gratitude and love for him. The profound effect that Avadhut Bhagwan Ram has had on my life is something much more pervasive and subtle. It has to do with his profound humility, his Christ-like presence that enabled him to suffer with grace the unceasing demands of his followers. Whenever I try to sum up the essence of what he taught me—not through his words but through his very presence—the following words come to me. They are my own, born out of my experience of the Avadhut: There is no religion higher than Truth, and there is no Truth higher than Compassion.

The Dance of Sri Vidya, the Path of Fulfillment

Following my experiences with Avadhut Bhagwan Ram I felt totally free of the need or desire for the living presence of a guru. Yet the higher self has a logic of its own. Gurus continue to manifest in my life as reflections of a continually expanding inner world. The current example of this is my relationship with Dr. N. Prahlad Sastry, or Amritananda, an adept and guru in the Sri Vidya tradition, one of the oldest and most respected Mother Goddess lineages in all of India. Amritananda is a former nuclear physicist who abandoned the world of defense contracts in order to find the original source of power in the Divine Mother. He and his wife, Annapurna Devi, together founded Devipuram, an ashram in the beautiful countryside outside Vishakapatnam in Andhra Pradesh, where they built a temple in the shape of a Sri chakra that houses the goddess Sri Rajarajeshwari ("Ruler of Rulers") and her 108 protectress goddesses, all sculpted in life-size forms.

The Sri chakra is the symbol used to represent the goddess in the Sri Vidya tradition. A series of intersecting triangles, it can be made in two or three dimensions, as either a yantra (a geometric diagram) or a three-dimensional, pyramidal *meru,* or "mountain." Both represent the goddess Sri in union with her consort. The downward-pointing triangles represent female energy, while those pointing upward represent male energy. The point at the center represents the starting point of creation, the point from which springs the entire universe. Simply stated, this tantric path involves the

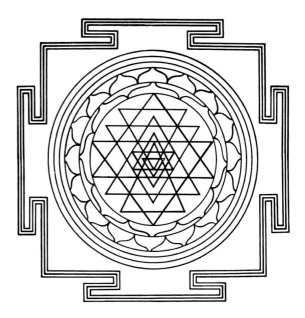

The central image of Sri Vidya is the Sri yantra or Sri chakra, symbolizing the entire cosmos as comprised of the intersection of male and female energies.

interplay of male and female energy on three levels: on the cosmic level, where the entire universe is understood as the body of the goddess; on the social level, in the attempt to realize the utopian dimensions of existence through loving relationships with others (recognizing the goddess in others); and finally, on the personal level, in realizing the goddess within the self as residing in the body, in the form of conscious awareness and power (shakti).

Having met Amritananda and Annapurna Devi over ten years ago, I have had the pleasure of watching Devipuram grow from the ground up. I have had the honor of dancing at the goddess's installation ceremony, and the joy of repeated visits to this enchanted abode. Owing to the grace of this "divine couple," my understanding of this vast tradition has grown into formal initiation into the practices of Sri Vidya. This has brought me into contact with an entire community of practitioners and goddess devotees throughout the world. Through my contact with this lineage I have increasingly experienced the presence of the goddess in everything around me.

Gurus and the Quest for Psychic Wholeness

In addition to these gurus there have been several other men in my life who have acted in varying capacities as spiritual teachers to me, including my first "wise old man" friend, my paternal grandfather, a small-scale farmer whose formal education never extended beyond the eighth grade. The simple stories my grandfather told me in my childhood, when I would sit by his side as he milked the cows, whetted my appetite for teachings handed down from ancestors. I also consider my former husband, to whom I was married for twenty years and who has always lived with the simplicity of a sadhu, to be an example in my life. And from a young age even my own son has imparted invaluable lessons to me. I am reminded here of the story of Yashoda, the mother of Krishna, who gets angry at her young son for stealing butter, but when she goes to punish him she sees the entire universe in his open mouth. There is a sense in which the guru is not limited to particular personalities but rather is an energy that one taps into, a state of mind in which one learns something about oneself from nearly every relationship.

However, being a feminist as well as a *sadhak* (religious practitioner), it once struck me as somewhat strange that the most important gurus in my life have been men rather than women. Having given it some consideration, I realize that this is exactly as it should be. Since I am myself a woman, it is the male aspect of my soul that, because of the socialization process, was originally unconscious and largely unexpressed. My longing for the guru was the soul's longing for what Jung calls the animus, the complementary male figure that, when made conscious, leads to psychic wholeness. Each of my male gurus reflected back to me some part of my male self that sought to become a more conscious part of who I am.

What is even more interesting is that all of the male gurus I have described here have themselves been especially attuned to feminine energy, which means they had already integrated or were in the process of integrating their male and female sides. Ganesh Baba was notorious for favoring his female disciples. When his married disciples would get in marital disagreements, he would almost invariably take the woman's side. He once told me, "Some people think that women are equal to men. That's nonsense. They are greatly superior." As I understood it, this attitude on his part didn't mean that he felt women were innately or biologically superior but rather that in spite of the fact that most cultures treated women as second-class citizens, many of the values instilled in women were, in a spiritual sense, superior to those championed by dominant males.

Ganesh Baba's preference for women was in keeping with his namesake, the elephant-headed Ganesh, who is a real mama's boy, as the myths humorously point out. Once Ganesh and his brother Kartikeya were arguing over who loved their mother, the goddess Parvati, more. They agreed to have a race. Whoever could circumnavigate the whole world and return to her side first would be declared the winner. Kartikeya, who is slim and trim compared with the potbellied Ganesh, took off in a streak of light while Ganesh dawdled around. Just before Kartikeya got back to his mother's side, Ganesh leisurely walked around his mother once and declared himself the winner. He explained that his mother *is* his whole world—therefore there was no need to go anywhere!

Even Agehananda Bharati and Apa Pant, both much-traveled men of the world, displayed this search for integration in their devotion to the goddess as well as in their great affection and respect for the women in their lives. Finally, both Bhagwan Ram and Amritananda are Shakta gurus, initiates of the goddess. Both have attained the level of total identification with their deities. Before his death, Avadhut Bhagwan Ram, who had worshiped Kali in the form of Vindhya Vasini Devi, was known to his disciples as Ma Guru, a manifestation of the goddess herself.

I have also been extremely fortunate to have enjoyed the teachings, blessings, and company of many well-known female yogis and *siddhas* (accomplished saints), including kriya *yogini* Beenama of Banaras, Gayatri Devi of Ananda Ashram in Cohasset, Massachusetts, Mata Amritananda of Kerala, and Mother Meera of Talheim, Germany. As well, not all of my female gurus have been Hindu. One of the most inspiring wisewomen I have ever met is Grandmother Twyla Nitsche, a Seneca elder from Cataraugus, near Buffalo, New York. Her example teaches that there is no limit to what can be achieved in a single lifetime by the will of a strong woman, regardless of race or nationality. While there are those who would like to see all Native teachings kept secret and accessible only to Natives, what Twyla offers is a unique synthesis of traditional Native American teachings and the insights gleaned from a lifetime spent serving Mother Earth and her creatures, a vision Twyla shares with people of all backgrounds and nationalities. In Grandmother's presence I distinctly felt her to be a vital link between past and future, between her blood ancestors and her spiritual descendants, and I am immensely grateful for her courageous energy.

Another extraordinary female teacher in my life was Sister Khechok Palmo, a Tibetan Buddhist nun. In her early life she was Mrs. Freda Bedi, an English-born social worker who was first introduced to Tibetan Buddhism through her work with Buddhist monks in southeast Asia. She ran a school for Tibetan Buddhists in Dharamsala, and in the early 1960s founded Karma Drubgyud Darje Ling, the first refugee nunnery for women in India. After taking full vows in the Kagyu lineage she dedicated her life to Vajrayana teachings, lecturing on Tibetan Buddhism and continuing to support the Tibetan refugee community in India.

I met Sister Palmo through her friend and protégée Joanna Macey, a practicing Buddhist whose "Despair and Empowerment" work is the best possible tribute to the memory of this great spiritual mentor. Sister Palmo had come to give a lecture on Tantric Buddhism at Syracuse University in the fall of 1974, when Joanna was doing graduate work in the religion department and I, recently returned from India, was completing the final year of my bachelor's degree. Sister Palmo cut a most impressive figure, with her long maroon robes and shaved head, but most memorable were her large blue eyes—eyes of depth and compassion. Because in her earlier years Sister Palmo had been a close associate of my husband's late grandfather, the great Sanskrit scholar Dr. Raghuvira, she graciously consented to come to our tiny apartment for a simple vegetarian dinner, along with Joanna and my professor, the now-famous authority on world religions, Dr. Huston Smith. I felt a great deal of warmth from Sister Palmo as during the meal my husband and I told her of our guru in India, and of our association with the Vedanta guru Mataji Gayatri Devi, the great-grandniece of Swami

Vivekenanda, who for many years had been serving in the ashram founded by her uncle, Swami Paramananda. Sister Palmo was surprised to hear of Mataji and mentioned that, since she was going to be staying in the Boston area, she might try to meet Mataji.

The following Easter my husband and I went to stay for a few days in Mataji's ashram and, as fate would have it, Sister Palmo called and made an appointment to visit while we were there. I was excited at the prospect of seeing her again, and of witnessing the meeting of these two great women. At the time I was five months into my first pregnancy. The morning that Sister Palmo was to visit I attended morning prayers and meditation, followed by a hearty breakfast of pancakes. Upon returning to our room I fell suddenly ill with violent stomach cramps. I vomited and expelled everything out of my digestive system. After a half hour of agony I realized there was some regularity to the gripping pains, and then it hit me—I was going into early labor! I timed the contractions and found that they were five minutes apart. Frightened, I made my way, doubled over, to the kitchen of the ashram and reported what was happening. The women immediately lay me down in an adjacent room while they went to inform Mataji. Shortly afterward Sister Palmo arrived, and when she heard that I was ill she insisted on seeing me. Left alone in the room for some time, I had lain on my back in corpse asana, closed my eyes, and begun concentrating on each breath, trying to relax into the contractions whenever they came. I could hear voices in the distance nervously discussing which doctor to call. Instinctively I knew that if I were going to keep the child I was carrying I had to stay very calm and focused.

After about fifteen minutes Sister Palmo entered the room and sat down beside me. In the most reassuring voice I have ever heard she told me not to worry. She then took something out of her bag and, holding it in her hand, began quietly to chant a long prayer in Tibetan. I remember how softly the sounds enveloped and calmed me, deepening my state of meditation. While I have told this story many times since, what happened next never ceases to fill me with wonder. No sooner had she finished the entire prayer than the pains completely stopped. I slowly opened my eyes. Tears were running down my cheeks.

Without the slightest surprise at what had just happened she told me that I would be all right from here on out. She made me swallow a small bit of some substance—a powder of some kind—prasad (ritual offerings) that she had recently received from His Holiness the Karmapa, her spiritual guru and head of the Karma Kagyu, the Red Hat sect of Tibetan Buddhism. Then she called my husband into the room and instructed him to purchase some vitamin E supplements for my nerves. I have always remembered her words to him: "She is very much like I was. Very sensitive. Overly active intellectual women like us don't really have an easy time carrying a child."

Though Sister Palmo had clearly prevented a miscarriage, Mataji nonetheless insisted that I visit a doctor. In his examination, however, the doctor could find no trace whatsoever that anything was amiss. He seemed almost doubtful when I described the excruciating pains I had experienced! After my son, Kapil, was born, I sent Sister Palmo a birth announcement thanking her profusely for what she had done. In turn she sent me a wonderful blessing—a dharma name for Kapil given by His Holiness Karmapa. While Sister Palmo did not live for many years after that—it is said that she left her body while in sitting meditation—I have never forgotten her many gifts to me. Nor did I realize that our lives would have some things in common. In her earlier, premonastic life she too had married an Indian from whom she later amiably separated. Like myself, she had one son, but hers, Kabir Bedi, became a well-known movie star in India and Italy. Her former husband, Baba Bedi, a learned Sikh, went on to become a spiritual teacher with disciples in India and Europe—by coincidence, years later I gave a dance performance in Turin, Italy, sponsored by his devotees.

Sister Palmo was also very familiar with the world of Indian classical dance. The late dancer Protima Bedi was her daughter-in-law. Protima was a high-profile Odissi dancer who had the reputation of an outspoken feminist in her younger years and who later in life went on to found Nityagram, a dance school in Bangalore, founded on the traditional gurukul model.

Sister Palmo had encouraged me to write and introduce myself to Protima, but I never did and our paths never crossed; nonetheless for years I followed her career in the media with great interest. Therefore I was shocked to read in the Indian newspapers in the fall of 1998 that Protima had been killed in a huge landslide that buried an entire encampment of religious pilgrims in the Himalayas. At first I was horrified to imagine her death, alone in the dark in her flimsy tent, high up in the mountains. They never did find her body, for she and the other pilgrims were completely buried under several feet of rock. However, the more I thought of it the more apt it seemed that her dramatic life should have an equally dramatic ending. As painful as it must be for her family, from another point of view there is a kind of awesome beauty in her final exit—the tremendous power of nature overtaking her, reclaiming her as its own, an incredible act of physical union in which the Earth itself refused to give her back. Like Sita, the heroine of the Hindu epic Ramayana, who prayed for Mother Earth to open and take her home, I believe that on some level Protima too was ready to go—before her death it is said that she had shaved her head, had rid herself of all unnecessary possessions, and had been spending more and more time in the "abode of the gods," the Himalayan mountains. The pilgrimage tour she was on was headed for Mount Kailash, the place where, according to Hindu myth, Lord Shiva and his consort Parvati are forever engaged in their dance of creation and destruction. Anyone who takes the long and arduous pilgrimage to that holy destination earns liberation. I like to believe that Protima was granted a shortcut.

The older I get the more my connection to Sister Palmo means to me. It is an archetypal theme in Indian mythology that Indian dancers, when they are tired of the world, shave their heads and become Buddhist nuns. With both Sister Palmo and her daughter-in-law as my role models, I am aware that my life is not over yet.

Extraordinary events such as this notwithstanding, it has been through much more "ordinary" women that I have felt the continual presence of feminine divinity in my life. Women like Sarojini Ma of Hyderabad, and countless other women I have known and loved in India and in other parts of the world, have sustained me in my spiritual life purely by their examples. It is through these living, breathing, hardworking women that the Mother Goddess has been made manifest in my day-to-day life. What amazes me the most, especially about Indian women, is that despite having been laden with so many responsibilities—many of them treated like second-class citizens from an early age, abused by their husbands and controlled by society—so many have not only survived with their humanity intact but actually thrived amidst the incredible challenges they face. Increasingly when people ask me why I keep traveling to India, I simply answer, "For the women. For what they teach me."

In the final analysis, whether I have sought to associate myself with enlightened women or have sought to integrate male energy within me through my male gurus, all paths lead home. I have traveled far and wide only to come full circle, back to the origin, to the Mother, who, in union with her consort, is none other than the totality I seek. Even in the world of dance my path eventually arrived on the doorstep of the Great Goddess herself. It is with the utmost regard that I refer to my present and last dance guru, Srimati A. Bala Kondalarao. After my first visit to India in 1972, I returned several times in subsequent years to study dance for three- to six-month periods. In 1981 my first guru, Master Natraj Ramakrishna, developed serious health problems and was unable to continue training me. While I studied for a while with my former *gurubhai* (guru brother) Kelam Sudarshan, in 1985 I traveled to Madras on the invitation of Dr. Vempati Chinnasatyam, India's most famous Kuchipudi dance master, whom I had met on tour in America. From the very beginning Master Chinnasatyam put me under the care and direction of Bala, his seniormost disciple and assistant.

I consider it no accident that I first met Bala in Kuchipudi village, the birthplace of this classical dance style, where she and Master Chinnasatyam were conducting a state Kuchipudi dance teacher's training course. After all, the patroness deity and resident of the oldest temple in Kuchipudi village is Bala Tripurasundari, one of the forms of the Great Goddess, whose name literally means "the eternally youthful goddess whose beauty illumines the three realms." (Bala Tripurasundari is also the goddess of Sri Vidya.) Her particular mantra, *aim*

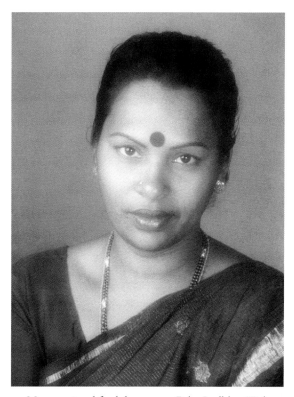

My present and final dance guru, Bala. I call her "Bala Tripurasundari," Goddess of the Three Worlds, the patroness deity of Kuchipudi dance. Photograph by B. K. Agarwal.

klim sauh, is one of the most important—and potent—of all invocations in the goddess-worshiping traditions of India. Whenever I write to my dance teacher I refer to her by this sacred name, but until recently I did not know that when I equate her with the goddess of Kuchipudi village, I am not alone. It turns out that she has been affectionately addressed as such even by members of the traditional dance families of Kuchipudi.

In a remarkable coincidence, it turns out that Bala's full name is very close to that of my late beloved devadasi teacher, Venkataratnama. Venkataratnama's name was Annabathula (family surname) Buli Venkataratnama, or "Vishnu's little jewel," while Bala's full name is Annakula (family surname) Buli Venkatabala, or "Vishnu's little goddess." Neither of these is a common name in South India. When I pointed this out to Bala, even she was surprised, and said, "Perhaps it was her love for you that led you to me."

From the first moment I saw Bala I thought she was the most graceful woman I had ever met. Each of her movements, such as the simple act of walking across the room, folding a piece of cloth, or picking up the telephone, takes on the qualities of a dance. Her honest and animated expressions combine with her grace to create an original and stunning presence. Her charisma is based not on external qualities conforming to some predetermined ideal but on an inner self-possession born of experience.

Bala's appearance and her direct, no-nonsense manner immediately struck me as completely different from the usual sophisticated urban style of dancers with whom I had previously come into contact. Because she is neither fair nor Aryan-featured, nor is she saccharin-tongued like so many of the city girls who inhabit the dance world, I immediately presumed she had grown up in a village, which turned out not to be the case at all. Now I realize that what I was responding to was her unusual strength and self-possession, a commanding confidence instilled in her by a solid cultural and family background thoroughly steeped in traditional values, yet flexible enough to keep an open and generous attitude toward new people and experiences and the world at large. Bala is the consummate teacher. She handles each student according to her or his individual personality; she is sometimes strict, sometimes playful, but always has one goal in mind—to bring out the potential within each person to best serve the art. While so many of the more famous dancers in India have inflated egos, thinking they have "mastered" the dance, Bala sees the Kuchipudi tradition as an inexhaustible ocean in front of which one cannot help but remain humble. At the same time, years of discipline have enabled her to effortlessly embody high standards in both her personal and professional lives so, as she says, she does not have to bow her head in front of anyone.

Like Venkataratnama, if ever anyone was born to dance it was Bala. From the age of five she knew her life's destiny and informed her parents of her intention to become a dancer. What is most extraordinary is that they took her seriously! Her father repeatedly asked her if she felt able to make the sacrifices necessary to achieve her goal. When she assured him that she did, he set out to find the best possible teacher for her. A few years later he and his wife and daughter traveled from their small town to the city of Madras. After a few visits they left Bala, at the age of nine, in the permanent care of Master Chinnasatyam, who raised her amidst his own family.

As she grew up she took on more responsibility at the Kuchipudi Arts Academy, serving as right hand to Master Chinnasatyam for over twenty-five years. For more than fifteen years she was the head teacher at the academy, and in that capacity taught many of the leading dancers in the current generation of the Kuchipudi art. The long list of her students includes many film stars; hundreds of dance teachers throughout India and abroad, including several from the traditional families of Kuchipudi; and even Master Chinnasatyam's own son and heir apparent, Ravi. In an interview conducted in 1989, Master Chinnasatyam told me that Bala is Ravi's guru. Bala told me the story of how Master did not want his son to become a dancer, so Ravi used to come to her for secret lessons. It was during the staging of the Chandalika dance drama, when Ravi made his debut dressed as one of the young girls, that Master wondered who the new dancer was and found out it was his son. From that point on Master Chinnasatyam had to recognize his son's talent.

Bala also came to play many of the lead characters in Vempati Chinnasatyam's Kuchipudi dance dramas, including *Rukmini Kalyanam* (The Marriage of Rukmini), and Chandalika, Tagore's classic story of an outcaste woman who offers water to Gautama Buddha. Bala traveled around the world twice, performing in over one hundred cities in seven countries over a ten-year period. But at the height of her performing career she took a radical step, relocating from Madras to Vishakapatnam in order to join her husband and "prove that a dancer can also live a family life." After serving for eleven years as the principal of the Kuchipudi Kalakshetra in Vishakapatnam, a branch institute of Vempati Chinnasatyam's Kuchipudi Arts Academy, in 1996 she founded her own institute, the Kuchipudi Kalakendra. Today she is increasingly gaining recognition throughout India as one of the leading teachers in the Kuchipudi tradition, and as a choreographer whose sophisticated dance compositions are infusing the Kuchipudi style with a renewed spirit of *bhakti*, or "devotion."

Having been her disciple for more than fifteen years now, I owe Bala the greatest debt for revealing to me what it really means to make dance my sadhana. To learn classical Indian dance is to take on a discipline that is at once difficult and rewarding, in my case one that appears at various times as a curse as much as a blessing. It is a blessing for all the insights I have gained and progress I have made, for the physical fitness and mental satisfaction of seeing ever more deeply into a particular art form over the course of a lifetime, and for the opportunity to make a contribution, however small, toward understanding between cultures.

My study of dance also sometimes feels like a curse because it demands so much on all levels. Every part of my body has been sore at one time or another. While dance certainly keeps me in shape, after a while I realized that I no longer have a choice whether or not to continue: If I stop not only does my entire body hurt, but I experience an incredible nagging guilt as well—all those years of training gone to waste! Dance is also an expensive undertaking. In earlier years I worked a variety of menial jobs in order to make enough money to return to India, only to spend long, lonely months undergoing various kinds of deprivations, illnesses, and inconveniences in order to learn a few more dances. I have actually gone hungry for the art on many occasions.

In fact, most Indians could never imagine the degree of sacrifice that westerners undergo in order to learn traditional arts in India. I have innumerable friends who have studied music or dance in India and each has his or her own harrowing tales to tell. When one comes from the comfortable life of the West, the spartan and sometimes downright unhealthy living conditions, the changes in cuisine, and the demands of a guru-student relationship all require a highly adaptable personality. For women it is especially difficult to live in India, as the image of western women in India is a highly distorted one. The majority of Indians, men and women alike, fantasize that we are sexually "free" and available, hence any nonconformist behavior on our part only confirms our suspect character. We have to live very circumspectly, constantly aware of how our actions come across to others. Of course, many Indians travel to the West, away from home and family, but they do so for different reasons. Most are extremely well-off, and I know of very few who travel to America or Europe to study the traditional arts or to learn anything about the

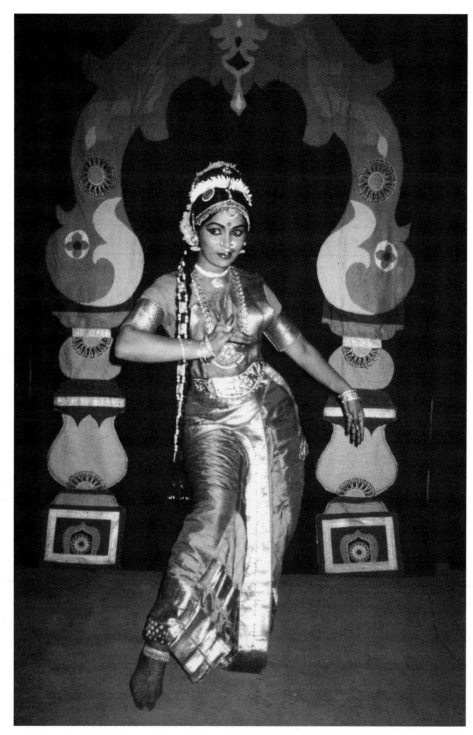

Bala in the role of Rukmini. One of Master Chinnasatyam's Kuchipudi dance ballets, Rukmini Kalyanam *(The Marriage of Rukmini), enacts the story of Lord Krishna's battle with Rukmini's selfish brother in order to win her hand in marriage. Rukmini was one of Bala's most famous roles during two world tours with Master's troupe.*

culture. In the West they are largely free to carry on with their way of life without being stared at, questioned, and judged.

In a sense my involvement in the art of Indian dance has sentenced me to a life of eternal displacement. In India I was and always will be somewhat alien, and because of India I have often felt like something of an outsider in my own culture. But despite all this, from the beginning I felt that I could never turn my back on India or the dance. I always joke that there is no such thing as quitting dance. When dance is finished with me, I am sure it will let me know.

Bala understands better than anyone both what I have sacrificed and what I have gained. Perhaps that is why she has encouraged me to persevere no matter what obstacles come in my way, just as she has done. By so doing I have come to realize that the lessons I have learned in the dance basically apply to my life as a whole: lessons regarding the development of will and inner strength; the courage to correct one's mistakes, to trust in superior guidance, to believe in something greater than oneself, to sacrifice in order to achieve one's ideals.

In Bala's class we don't use mirrors. The guru alone is our mirror, and sometimes it is difficult to face what one sees there. When after doing a short sequence she tells me that I have to lean farther forward, lift my leg higher, stretch my arms out more fully to the side, lift my elbows, keep my eyes focused to the front, and smile, I want to curse, grit my teeth, or cry out, "Aren't I doing anything right?" Instead, I have to bear it and try my best to do exactly as she says, otherwise I know that she will make me do it over and over until I get it right. (Or worse yet, she won't continue telling me!)

Sometimes my own stubbornness amazes me. How attached I can be to my own way of doing something! Even when she tells me a certain movement is wrong, I sometimes don't want to listen. I like the way it feels, I like the way I think I am doing it, and it bruises my ego to think I have to do it another way. There have even been times when, in response to her critique, my body engages in passive resistance—it just refuses to do what she wants me to. My mind observes my own stupidity, what my body is doing, and it too stands back and watches: What will happen if I just ignore her? This inner struggle takes place in a matter of seconds. I look at Bala and wonder if she knows what's going on, and of course she does. She knows very well. I cannot hide anything from the mirror. I see her planning her next move and wonder what she will say or do to get me to realize that I have to submit to this discipline, to give up my delusions and believe in her judgment, to put my fate in her hands. We stare into each other's eyes—I am like a defiant child with her mother. I know Mother loves me, but how is she going to show it? By letting it pass, or by forcing her will on me? By gentle explanation, or with shouts? Every day when I enter the class I lay myself on the line again; I face the same fears: Can I do it? Should I even try?

This is dance as therapy, and Bala is the supreme practitioner working not only with my mind but with my entire being. With her I have to learn to walk all over again. The struggle itself is a blessing. To challenge oneself and grow beyond one's self-imposed limits is the empowering nature of art as sadhana, spiritual practice. Although I cannot dedicate myself as totally as my guru Bala has, and hence will never approach her level of attainment, there is no loss for me, because where my dance ends hers begins. When she dances, so does my soul. My first guru, Natraj Ramakrishna, once presented me with a title, a typical way of honoring a student. The title he gave me was "Natya Kala Kaumudi," which literally translates as "the moonlight of Indian dance." If I am moonlight, Bala is the sun. I am more than satisfied to live in my guru's shadow, and reflect some of her light.

My experience of Indian classical dance, then, is the most perfect expression of my relationship to India—a give and take in which I try to offer something back in return for all that I have received. But the dance is also the most perfect expression of my individual experience of who I am—the dance between my inner self and my ever-changing outer identity, which finds itself in relationship to others and the world.

Coomaraswamy, an early-twentieth-century art historian and philosopher, captured this sense in a poetic verse in his now-classic treatise on Indian art, *The Dance of Siva:*

When the Actor beateth the drum,
Everybody cometh to the show.
When the Actor collecteth the stage properties
He abideth alone in His happiness.

But for me this experience comes before, not after, the dance.

Standing backstage alone, it is dark. I can see the stage, dimly lit, waiting for me. I smell the burning incense as it drifts from the altar of Nataraja, Lord of the Dance. I hear the rustling of the people in the audience and feel their anticipation. Anxiety lies just beneath the surface calm of my mind, for under the stage lights there is nowhere to hide. Although I am wearing an elaborate costume, makeup, and jewelry, I may as well be naked, for if the performance is not just a show, even the dancer's soul will be exposed. The time has come to face the mirror.

Taking a deep breath, I let go and offer the results to Nataraja. I close my eyes and breathe a prayer: May this offering bring happiness, healing, and insight to all present. In a heartbeat my gurus are all with me: Master and Venkataratnama, Bala, and of course Ganesh Baba, the remover of all obstacles. In that moment I am finally at peace within myself. I am fully conscious, fully aware. I am not the costume, not the image that I am about to present, not even the body beneath the costume. But if I am not the body, not the drama, not even the soul about to be bared, who am I? I pray to gods and gurus to grant me the final awareness: I am the stillness at the center. I am the dance.

THREE

Stillness at the Center

The Yoga of Indian Dance

Whether one is a performer of the art or a member of the audience, an understanding of the principles that inform Indian dance is necessary in order to fully experience its depths and nuances. In this chapter I discuss Indian dance in terms of its classical form within the tradition as well as my own understanding of the dance as yoga, for in my experience with both disciplines I have become aware of the ways in which they parallel and sometimes overlap each other.

There are important differences, and equally important similarities, between Indian classical dance and yoga. While yoga is inner oriented, dance is oriented to an external audience; yet both disciplines involve integrating inner, subjective experience with outer, objective form. Both operate on all levels of our being, engaging the three bodies—the physical, the psychic, and the spiritual or causal—yet in neither yoga nor dance are these three levels understood as separate from each other. They are instead hierarchical and interpenetrating: the spiritual encompasses all levels, and the psychic both translates the transcendent into image and offers it access to the physical. On the physical level, by contrasting movement with stasis in creatively varied patterns, Indian classical dance mirrors the passage of time against the backdrop of eternity, and through rhythm it hypnotically connects the dancer and audience on deep levels of consciousness. On the psychic plane, through the projection of potent images dance works in a manner similar to the visualization techniques of yoga. According to the classical tradition, dance, performed as an offering to the gods, is like yoga, a sadhana through which the highest spiritual goal can be realized. The goal is described as *moksha,* liberation, or freedom from all individual limitation.

However, just as in yoga, in all the classical arts of India, whether it be performing arts such as dance and drama or fine arts such as sculpture and painting, this freedom is attained only through discipline, not only of the body but of the psyche and spirit as well. For this reason dance, like yoga, has been handed down from guru to student in a practical system in which teachings are passed on orally. While the physical postures as well as the general theory and specific techniques of dramatic production are directly based on Sanskrit treatises, the most authoritative being the *Natya Sastra,* most traditional dancers did not actually read the *Natya Sastra,* although they were undoubtedly familiar with specific verses of the text. The knowledge contained in the Sastras was always an applied knowledge—understood and passed on in a practical way.

It is in the modern period that the written text has taken on new importance. Today a particular dance style is determined to be "classical" relative to its adherence to the *Natya Sastra.* All styles of Indian classical dance must follow the basic principles of this text. According to the *Natya Sastra,* all dance falls under three categories: *nritta, nritya,* or *natya.* In nritta, or "pure dance," the dance poses and gestures are entirely abstract; hence, the emphasis is on the physical form. In nritya, or "lyrical dance," bodily stance and movement, hand gestures known as *hastas* or *mudras,* and facial expressions are used to convey the meaning of the lyrics of the accompanying song; hence, the symbolic or psychic elements are given importance. In natya, or "dramatic dance," *abhinaya*—expression—predominates. Abhinaya is the most subtle aspect of Indian dance, and is what determines its aesthetic value. Anyone can learn to imitate certain physical movements, but abhinaya is the magical component of drama.

The *Natya Sastra* lists four kinds of abhinaya: *angika,* or bodily stance and movement; *vachika,* or expression of the voice through speaking and singing as well as through the music itself; *aharya,* or costumes and decoration; and *satvika,* or the subtle conveyance of emotion through feeling. There is often a thin line between nritya and natya because both involve abhinaya, but whereas nritya remains symbolic, natya may include sections in which the dancer acts out in a more realistic way certain episodes from the Hindu myths described through poetry and song. Reflecting upon what the *Natya Sastra* is conveying about the relationship of dance and drama, one might say that the magic of abhinaya, the essence of drama, is what gives dance its deeper significance.

Among all the dance traditions of the world, the Indian classical dance tradition is singularly "self" conscious: it reflects upon its own nature, its inner workings and higher principles. The *Natya Sastra* offers a mythological account of drama having been created by the gods themselves. Drama is equated with revelation, and hence is referred to as the fifth Veda. Expounding upon the processes of dramatic creation, which reflect as well on cosmic creation, the *Natya Sastra* gives instructions not only for creating abstract physical form but also for symbolically depicting various classes of human and mythological characters. Finally, drama is spiritual in its intent. Through its myths and symbols a recurrent and consistent theme is played out—the theme of desire bonding the Absolute and the limited, the Divine and the human—and directing the incarnation of infinite spirit into finite form.

Developing the Physical Form

What is most unique about Indian classical dance is the stillness that is integrated into its movement. This stillness, at the heart of what I call the yoga of Indian dance, is easy to apprehend from the outside but very difficult to realize, both physically and as an inner state of consciousness. In its basic form, Indian dance creates the effect of a series of still poses *(karanas)* that gracefully flow one into the next. (This is particularly true of the South Indian styles, with their bent-knee positions.) Taken individually, these poses resemble the classical sculptures carved on the walls of Hindu temples, and similarly incorporate aspects of various yoga asanas. The still pose is an ideal form one is seeking to attain, while the *laya* or internal sense of rhythm determines the flow: it is the grace with which the dancer reaches the stillness. The poses move in sequence following the drum and the *nattuvangam*, a series of abstract syllables recited by the guru or dance director as he plays the *talam,* small brass symbols. The guru thus leads both the music and the dance, sitting with the musicians on the side of the stage. The nattuvangam actually directs the dancer's footwork patterns. When recited rapidly the nattuvangam has an interesting sound quality in and of itself, something like scat singing in jazz.

While its association with the cosmic dancer, Lord Shiva Natraj, indicates that Indian dance is deeply rooted in ancient techniques of invoking ecstatic states of consciousness, over time the art has developed in such a way that whatever ecstasy remains is highly controlled. In fact, the kind of ecstasy that is invoked by Indian dance might more accurately be called *enstasy,* the inner, blissful state attained through yogic meditation. Reaching such a state through the dance is both a long process and a rare achievement. First the physical technique must be practiced until it can be performed nearly automatically, and the hand gestures and various expressions must be learned like a language. Only then can the dancer begin to experience the stillness at the center: more subtle levels of energy and a higher state of consciousness in the midst of movement. In this way Indian dance is comparable to western ballet, which looks graceful and simple but which actually requires years of training to master.

Like ballet, both yoga and Indian dance involve conformity to an ideal form determined by tradition and governed by predetermined rules. In the case of Indian dance it is often stated that, in order to conform to tradition, the individuality of the artist has to be relinquished to the art form. The notion that one has to empty the self in order to submit to discipline is an idea that is much repeated within Indian culture.

As a westerner, I understand the concept of self-discipline in a different way. I understand aesthetic and spiritual development not only as a process of increasing universality or identification with a collective, and even cosmic, consciousness, but also in terms of what Carl Jung referred to as increasing individuation, a process by which the individual becomes more uniquely herself even as she finds her place in the whole. These two processes need not work against each other, though working with both calls for psychic agility as we freely move between the two poles of individuality and universality. The classical arts of the world's great wisdom traditions demonstrate that these poles are forever in communion with each other through the language of symbol and myth.

Invoking the Psychic Realm

All Indian dance takes its themes from Hindu mythology. Dance is an integral part of the larger tradition of drama in India, which is understood as a sacred activity akin to the sacrificial fire, a sacred ritual of Vedic Hinduism. A verse in the *Natya Sastra* states that the gods gather around the sacred stage of drama like they gather around the sacrificial fire. This verse indicates the central position of drama in ancient Indian culture, granted for its power to invoke divine presence in the midst of human society.

Indian drama gives full expression and religious sanction to human emotions and desires by demonstrating that life on earth is a reflection of higher transcendent realms, especially *svarga loka*, the realm of the gods. In svarga loka, the heavenly realm, the many gods and goddesses of the Hindu pantheon interact in a series of relationships that reflect all-too-human concerns, for these relationships are more often than not erotic. The clear-cut distinction between the secular and the sacred, between human and divine, a major hallmark of Judeo-Christian and Islamic monotheism, is totally undermined by the polytheistic Hindu pantheon and its polymorphous proclivities. Krishna has sixteen thousand concubines, his favorite being Radha, another man's wife. Kama, the god of love, disturbs Shiva's meditation with his flower arrows, causing him to fall in love with Parvati. When Shiva burns Kama to ashes, his wife Kamakshi, "She Whose Eyes Fulfill All Desire," brings him back to life. While Indian dance and drama display the entire gamut of human emotion, in the dance the erotic sentiment is by far the most popular. Even within the temples, where devadasis offered their dance before the deity, it was explicitly understood that the dance represented an offering of sexual intercourse. Within the Hindu worldview all areas of human life were seen as essential parts of the whole, and sexuality, in both its erotic and reproductive aspects, was understood as a reflection of the Divine.

In the yogic traditions all such dramas, both human and divine, are understood as taking place within the self. The eros, or creative interaction, between freedom and limitation, between energy and matter—also known as Shiva and Shakti, the archetypal male and female principles—give rise not only to the whole human drama but to the entire cosmos. This is divine eros, passion between humanity and the gods. From a psychological perspective we can conceptualize svarga loka as a projection of the human psyche, the realm of consciousness that mediates between the universe of Absolute Spirit and limited physical human existence. Within the psyche, gods, goddesses, and other beings act out the archetypal themes that lie at the heart of human existence.

This interaction between humans and gods is well displayed in the oldest and most famous dance drama of the Kuchipudi tradition, the Bhama Kalapam. This dance drama tells the story of Satya Bhama and her relationship to the Supreme Lord and Divine Lover, Krishna. (Satya Bhama is Krishna's most proud and beautiful wife.) The dance opens with the heroine, Bhama, introducing herself as the treasured daughter of the great King Satyajit and, for possessing unequaled beauty and intelligence, as Krishna's favorite concubine. According to mythology Krishna, an incarnation of Vishnu the Preserver, has eight wives and sixteen thousand paramours, so the dramatic tradition associated with him often includes themes centering on jealousy or competitiveness between women. In this play the heroine becomes angry when she hears that Krishna has given a *parijata* flower to Rukmini, his first wife. Satya Bhama in turn demands that Krishna plant an entire tree in her yard. He does as she requests, but the flowers from the tree fall only next door in Rukmini's yard. Bhama gets upset and confronts Rukmini, asking how Rukmini is getting the flowers from Bhama's tree. Finally, Sage Narada explains to her that the parijata flower will come only to those whose love for God is truly selfless.

The central theme of this drama is the love between the human and the Divine. According to the tradition, Bhama represents the egoistic self who, overcome with passionate longing, demands that she alone be graced with the special attention and favor of God. Intoxicated as much with her self as with her Lord, she finally has to submit her ego to the realization that without her Lord she is lost. In the end Bhama realizes the foolishness of her egoism, and that it is the Supreme Lord Krishna, not she, who is truly great.

In this drama Satya Bhama, chastened by Krishna's love, is forced into a state of humility. However, beyond this simple message about selfless love the drama has a more complex theme; there is a sense in which the humanity of Satya Bhama is also celebrated. The passion Bhama feels for Krishna is not only her weakness. It is also her strength. Because of her love for him, imperfect as it is, Krishna also favors Bhama: God longs for the human as much as the human longs for him; it is only egoism that prevents one from realizing the infinite love that is always present. The higher or transcendent lesson of the Bhama Kalapam is that overidentification with the ego only leads to separation from our true goal, which is union with the Absolute, but for the heroine that lesson is achieved only through *kama* or eros, the passion of her love.

It is one thing to understand the moral of the story, but it is another thing altogether to actually experience it. Dance and drama seek to invoke the divine realm on earth—not merely to represent it in a symbolic sense but to give it body, to make it actually come to life on the human stage. Dance is the ritual means used to make this happen. To witness such a performance under the spotlights of a theater or under the stars of an open-air performance on an Indian summer night is to experience the presence of gods on earth.

To enter into the role of a god or goddess on stage is an even more transforming experience, but one that is not without its difficulties. As a western woman I have had challenges relating to some of the mythological portrayals of the dance. It is here that the issue of gender relations and sexual politics enters into the dancer's relationship to her art. Reflecting dominant societal values, many dances portray the feminine in a subservient position to a male hero or god figure. I am not the only dancer who sometimes has great trouble relating to a dance in which a woman pouts and pleads with her lover not to abandon her for another woman, even if the meaning is primarily symbolic. There are certain dances that I have no interest in performing and others that I am able to play with, to interpret to my own satisfaction without compromising my self-respect. For there are some dances, including some contemporary compositions centering on the goddess, where women emerge as strong figures in their own right. As many Indian dancers will admit, it is difficult to project a theme on the stage without identifying with it to some extent in your own life. As someone born in the West I am perhaps more easily empowered to express my individuality in relationship to the art form, although many Indian women today are doing the same.

While onstage the dancer must be able to carry the audience's projections. Thus, a certain level of maturity is necessary in the dancer, and the right audience is also called for. The characteristics of a cultured audience are prescribed in the *Natya Sastra*. The audience should be capable of understanding the more subtle aspects of the dance themes and able to accept the performance on all levels. The offering of dance on the stage is like an act of intercourse that takes place between the dancer and the audience—it is a psychospiritual relationship in which the dancer exposes her vulnerability even as she reveals her inner beauty and power.

In any dance program, from the moment I enter the stage I can feel the audience's mood. In the beginning I can feel their breathless expectancy, like that of a lover waiting in excited anticipation. In this relationship I am in the active role. The audience expects me to take command, to carry them away to another world, to allow them to momentarily forget themselves. But at the same time in forgetting their cares I want them to remember something much more basic, something so simple they may have forgotten that they ever knew it: that the dance they perceive on the stage is taking place within their own conscious awareness. The awe with which the audience regards the dance is the awe with which we should approach each other, and all of life. This is the gift of the dance: eros, consciousness on its most intimate level, a mutual recognition of our interconnectedness. An expression of our essential blissful nature, eros binds us to each other and to this earth, to creation as a whole.

Embodying the Spirit

The spirit lives through flesh and blood, heart and mind. True spirituality manifests through the physical *and* the psychic: only when they truly come together can transcendence take place.

In all the years I have been performing there have been only a few times that I have actually been able to completely lose myself in the dance. It usually seems necessary to keep at least a part of my consciousness focused on the mechanics, the actual techniques necessary to maintain the form of the dance. And yet, even while concentrating on what needs to be done it is still possible to experience an intense high from the dance. This happens when all of the individual components of the dance seem to lock into place, and the dance begins to flow in a continuous and effortless stream. It really does seem as if a higher power enters in and charges the movement with energy, and the dancer is carried along as if floating on a powerful current. It is possible to feel the effects of that "flow" on the audience. There have been times when the excitement of the audience reflects back to me in waves so strong that I break into goosebumps while I am dancing. Unlike the experience of yoga, this is a kind of ecstasy that exists not entirely within the performer, but between the performer and the audience. Dance *is* eros.

Indian dance is of course not the only kind of traditional dance that demonstrates this kind of power. In fact, my experiences with African and Afro-Caribbean dance have made me feel that they afford an even more immediate gratification—certainly to the dancer, and perhaps to the audience as well. While both Indian and African dance are extremely grounded or earthbound (compared with ballet and modern dance), Indian dance is more sublime in the literal sense—it involves a complete sublimation of the kind of sexual energy that gives such powerful life to African dance. Dance reflects the basic values of a culture. Reflecting a culture that remained largely tribal based, African dance celebrates nature as being at the heart of culture, whereas Vedic culture "colonized" nature and subjugated tribalism early on. In attempts to tame nature, sexuality is the first arena subject to control. As a result, in comparison with that of African and Caribbean societies, Indian sexuality in general is highly circumscribed and overlaid with layers of religious meaning and control. Like tantric yoga, Indian dance invokes sexual eroticism in order to channel it upward in the spirit of transcendence. Yet the process evokes its own kind of ecstasy.

Another interesting comparison between cultures, on the psychic level, has to do with the invocation of specific energies through dance. While Indian dance invokes the archetypal energies of the Hindu gods and goddesses, African dance traditions call forth personified energies or deities called *orishas*. African dance can quickly induce altered states of consciousness, enabling the orishas to inhabit the bodies of the dancers. In India the mainstream culture views such possession as highly dangerous. With few exceptions, such types of ritual today are considered folk practices involving "lower" nature spirits, and are performed mainly by lower-caste persons. Within Indian classical culture (that is, the arts developed by the literary elite) it is mainly through various forms of religious drama that the major deities can in any sense inhabit human bodies, and even then the gods are very controlled. According to Indian culture, it is only through the control of divine energy that humans can attain the ideal embodied in the form of a "classical" art.

What is interesting to me is the way in which the ideal form is adapted by the individual, even today in India, where conformity is still the rule. A dance movement taught to several students, all of whom eventually master the movement, will appear unique when performed by each student. On the physical level, the ideal exists in theory alone; the movement can manifest only imperfectly through its actual application. Whether it is yoga or dance, as long as we remain physical beings the ideal remains something for which we are always striving rather than something that can be actually fully attained. Instead of bemoaning that fact one can accept the limitations inherent in embodied human state and, when engaged in any physical discipline, concentrate on the process of striving for the goal rather than reaching the goal as an end in itself.

Yet, since the very concept of an ideal or transcendent realm is translated through the mental body (the psychic realm), as humans we are capable of attaining the ideal on that level. It is not only in the artistic realm that the creativity of the imagination comes into play. Cosmology, mythology, philosophy, and even the sciences are all, in a sense, "imaginary." As expressions of the human capacity for conceptualization and abstraction, they are all functions of the psyche. Whenever humankind reflects upon the nature of self and the universe it is the psychic body that comes into play. Our limitations are purely physical, while our subtle bodies are as agile and unlimited as our imaginations. It is when the subtle body is projected through the physical that the dance becomes truly powerful. In this way the subtle body or psychic consciousness mediates between the realm of the spirit—pure or universal consciousness—and the physical. Consciousness is the common factor, and it is consciousness alone that pervades all realms—from the most subtle to the gross. It is truly consciousness that dances.

How can we practically realize this? Put most simply, it means that in striving for an ideal, any ideal, we must identify primarily with subtle human capabilities. To realize the unlimited character of our true nature we must give up our predominant identification with the physical realm. However, this does not mean to neglect or denigrate the physical; in fact, it means quite the opposite. Through disciplines such as yoga and dance we can come to honor the body as sacred, the playhouse of the spirit. At the same time we are free to transcend, through the psyche, the limitations we encounter on the physical plane. There is no question that the psychic realm influences the physical; it is only our limited perspective that gives the illusion of their separation. According to the Hindu perspective, the subtle (consciousness) gives birth to the gross (matter). Matter itself is merely "condensed" consciousness.

For this reason, I consider neither dance nor yoga as a primarily physical discipline. Both are, first and foremost, expressions of energy. If dance is spiritual it is so because through it we can transparently perceive the movement of energy in the body. All dance is the play between the physical form, which is limited, and the infinite spirit, which is free. The stillness at the center is where body and spirit meet. Their interplay is the eros of Indian classical dance.

FOUR

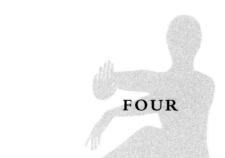

The Dance of Yoga
The Sixty-Four Yogini Asanas

In the marriage of Indian dance and yoga, what dance brings to yoga is its essentially feminine nature; in other words, its eroticism. Here *eroticism* does not refer to sexuality in a narrow sense but rather points to a more expansive conception of universal relatedness. As the primary creative principle, feminine energy draws things together, fosters connection, and manifests in the world as both passionate and compassionate love. In previous chapters I have spoken at length about the symbolic significance of the Indian dancer, who embodies these erotic aspects of creation and the world. It is important to know that yoga also acknowledges this feminine principle as central to its transcendent purpose. In the tantric formulations that form the theoretical basis of all schools of yoga within India, this feminine principle is called Kundalini.

Kundalini, the "serpent power," is conceived as a primordial energy that lies coiled and dormant at the base of the spine. With time and practice, she is believed to rise and pierce through the various energy plexuses *(chakras)* located along the spine. This is conceived of as an extremely subtle process, brought about by both physical and psychic techniques. If the goal is achieved Kundalini rises with a tremendous force, unlocking the doors of inner perception, unleashing pent-up energies, and breaking all boundaries, liberating the personality from all its previously held, limited categories of self-understanding. Finally, reaching the uppermost level and infusing the *sahasrara,* the thousand-petaled lotus located at the top of the skull, with her primal energy, the Kundalini shakti unites with her male counterpart

(Shiva, or Divine Consciousness) and liberation is achieved. This blissful state of inner mystical union is the ultimate goal of all yoga.

It is not coincidental that the tantric tradition, which developed the yogic chakra system, is also the oldest living goddess-worshiping religion in the world; at the heart of Indian metaphysics and spirituality lies the relationship between the body and feminine power. The image of the chakras constructs a subtle body of energy that enables the yoga practitioner to negotiate the relationship between the physical, psychic, and spiritual worlds within his or her own body, and between that body and the outer world.

In various tantric schools the chakra system also relates to the more symbolic philosophical and theological aspects of the Indian tradition. These stress the interrelationship of male and female, spirit and matter. The Sri Vidya system describes how each chakra is the site of a specific form of the goddess, who is seated in union with her male consort. These representations of union at each of the points are reflective of the overall mystical union of male and female energies that is the ultimate goal of yoga.

Despite the essential role of the feminine energy in this process, there is no doubt that yoga, as traditionally practiced in India, has primarily been defined as a male discipline. Mention the word *yogi* and the first thing that comes to mind is a half-naked, matted-haired holy *man*. In fact, the various forms of asceticism identified with yoga in India have long been contrasted with their opposite, the sexuality and fertility of women, aptly symbolized by the Indian dancer. And yet it has been the wisdom of Indian culture to recognize that opposites not only attract; they are somehow locked into an eternal dance of relatedness. In India the archetypes of the holy man and the temple dancer go together as naturally as Shiva and Shakti, each embodying the essence of male and female energies as well as their interrelationship. Asceticism and eroticism are the two magnetic poles that generate the highly charged electricity of Indian spirituality.

This interrelationship of male and female is a cosmic dance that takes place in all our lives, whether or not we practice yoga, whether or not we are aware of it. This dance takes place both in the external world, through the gendered, specifically male and female bodies we inhabit and the roles we play in relation to each other, as well as within ourselves, as we strive in various ways to achieve our own versions of psychic wholeness, to effectively balance our own male and female aspects. In Jungian terms, this is what the process of individuation is all about. Not only in yoga but in various spiritual traditions, both eastern and western, this dance presents itself as prelude to mystical union. And yet even within tantrism, the tradition that most explicitly and eloquently honors this union, with all we know about yogis, how little we ever hear about yoginis, their female counterparts.

Over time the yoginis have nearly disappeared from India, and we can hardly remember who they were. Yet ancient tantric manuscripts—which are only now, at the end of the twentieth century, being taken from dusty shelves, translated, and analyzed—offer ample evidence that there were once many yoginis in India. At the very least we know that yogini cults once flourished, and that women played major roles in these schools of tantrism, which celebrated the unity of the cosmos: nature, spirit, and body.

And yet it is true that despite all the texts, field information, and indigenous expertise available to us, scholars from India and the West are not yet able to definitively state who the yoginis actually were. In some texts they appear as mythological, semidivine figures, and in others as human beings. In some traditions the yoginis are promoted into full-fledged Mother Goddesses, while in folk legends they appear, like yogis, to straddle the boundaries of human and divine. To make things even more complex, they can appear as both benign and frightening. It seems that much does remain, and will continue to remain, up to human interpretation. If I were to speak strictly as a scholar I would have to conclude that nothing can be proven about who the yoginis *were,* and leave it at that. But as a practitioner of Indian spiritual disciplines I believe I *know* who the yoginis *are,* and who they might *be* for us, both today and in the future. If the yogini never existed we would have to create her. But since she (not one, but many) did exist, we now must rediscover her, to find her in our own re-creation, and in our truly spiritual re-creation of yoga and dance.

In the title of this book the *yogini's mirror* refers to the mirror that dance holds up to yoga, so that this formerly world-denying discipline can begin to recognize its complementary aspect here and now on earth. If yoga is about transcending death, dance is about embracing life. As yogis and yoginis, we must learn to do both.

Who, then, is the yogini we now rediscover? She is one who, like the yogi, seeks to overcome opposites. However, insofar as the yogi seeks to overcome opposites within, the yogini seeks to overcome opposites both within and without. She is as concerned with the world of creation as she is with the reality beyond death. And unlike the yogi who sits, stands, or lays down to practice a series of distinct yoga exercises, the yogini dances yoga from beginning to end. She weaves a tapestry that, by its very nature, transcends the opposition between spirit and matter—between the infinite and creation—and that dissolves those barriers which irreconcilably divide the world and alienate us from nature, God, and ourselves. The yogini is the energy of eros, the great coming together of self, world, and cosmos. She is conscious of her relations. In a real sense we are not re-creating her; it is she who re-creates us. Through her dance of yoga she is re-creating the world in her own image.

Bringing It Down to Earth

How can we know the yogini? How can we become her? In a most basic sense, this dance of re-creation begins with the body. Toward this end I offer in this chapter my sixty-four yogini asanas, the number sixty-four being an archetypal number associated in the Hindu tradition with the yoginis and their mystical powers. This is my own creative rendering; no text exists within the tradition prescribing these or any other hatha yoga asanas in association with yogini cults. In naming these the sixty-four yogini asanas I seek to symbolically reclaim the hatha yoga tradition for women's bodies.

But our efforts must not end with these asanas. Yoga is a physical discipline that moves in, through, and beyond the physical level as soon as consciousness becomes aware of itself. Consciousness is key. There are no limits as to where it can take you. In concrete terms, this means that yoga works precisely to the degree that you are aware you are practicing it. This does not mean becoming self-conscious in a negative sense, but instead becoming conscious of the self in its expanded dimensions. This might seem an easy task, but sometimes obstacles can stand in our way. We as humans (women especially, but not exclusively) have been made to feel self-conscious and even ashamed of our bodies. Therefore, much of yoga involves a cleaning out of our bodies and psyches and a clearing away of the physical and mental toxins and debris we have attracted through our individual and collective experiences. Yoga offers us a way to unplug from the narrow bounds of our physical identity, as dictated by our culture, and open up to other, expanded, levels of our being.

There is no question that yoga can help one to transform physically. For me, not only is there nothing wrong or selfish with striving to improve one's physical health and beauty; I believe it should be openly embraced as a basic responsibility to self and others. But why stop there? If we can let go of understanding ourselves as primarily physical beings, our very notions of health and beauty can be expanded so greatly that we begin to see the world in an entirely new way. When we begin to develop and recognize inner beauty, the beauty of the soul as well as the body, our confining cultural categories will begin to crack and we might be able to collectively liberate ourselves from the narrow judgments that have programmed us for so many centuries.

Therefore, if I could use only two words to describe both the means and goal of my hatha yogini practice they would be *expand* and *embrace*. Expand physically and mentally, emotionally, and spiritually. Expand as far as you can, and embrace all that you are, all that the world has to offer. Embrace not only the beauty but also that which has been rejected, whether it is in yourself or in someone else. For it is only by embracing that transformation can take place. Even if you ultimately need to let go, embrace, and *then* let go. This is distinct from the traditional formula for yoga, which might be stated as expand and transcend. In the past yoga has often been used as a way to escape one's limitations and problems, and the sorrows of the world. Yet the highest yogis will tell you that there is really no place to go. True transcendence can only take place in the here and the now. When we begin to open ourselves to all that we are and all that the world is; when we begin to recognize the depth of our relationship to others, and to honor the connections between ourselves and nature; when we begin to dance with the flow of the various interactions that constitute our larger reality, then yoga becomes more than a practice—it becomes the real thing, the dance of life.

If we want to dance our lives, then we can start by making our yoga a dance. My understanding and practice of yoga has from the beginning been inextricably linked to my practice of Indian dance. Several years ago I found that the two disciplines were naturally overlapping—for when I was totally involved in my yoga, I would find myself automatically making the asanas flow into each other, as if in a dance. Later I began to put various asanas together in series so that, like Surya Namaskar, the asanas could be repeated in cycles. These cycles end up at the same place they begin, and can be repeated as many times as one likes. It is also possible to vary the tempo at which the cycles are performed; the same asana can be performed in a vigorous way that energizes you, or in a slow, repetitive, and calming mode that releases all the tension in your body and mind.

Yogic Breathing

The practical starting point and most important component of yoga practice is the breath. The ability to regulate one's breath is the most basic level on which we are able to take control over our lives. Our dependence on air is the most fundamental fact of our existence. We can survive without food or water for days, but we can't live for more than a few minutes without air; yet breathing is the physiological function we most take for granted. The very idea that we should have to relearn how to breathe seems strange to most people, and yet it doesn't take long for those who try it to realize the benefits. Through increased oxygen intake not only does your body function more efficiently, but your emotions begin to calm and your mind becomes clearer and more focused. By linking breath and consciousness, we awaken inner awareness and begin to relate to the world in new and creative ways.

So we begin with the breath to apprehend that which is more subtle. Even in hatha yoga, which centers on asanas or bodily postures, it is not the physical but the subtle dimension of conscious awareness that we strive for. That means that when practicing an asana we should concentrate not only on the outer posture but, more important, on projecting consciousness inward to become increasingly aware of inner sensations associated with various parts of the body. Of course, to initially learn the asanas you must start with the outer form, the physical posture. But that is only the beginning. In order to visualize the internal realm, know that consciousness follows the breath. It is through awareness of the movement of breath inside the body that one can travel the inner world. This is why it is important for students of yoga to learn correct breathing patterns from the beginning.

While different branches of yoga have developed a variety of breathing exercises designed to affect consciousness in specific ways, the pranayama, or yogic breathing, that I practice is very simple: inhale/expand, exhale/contract. On the inhalation the lungs, like a balloon, fill with air, which causes the chest and abdomen to expand. When exhaling, consciously pull your abdominal muscles inward so that the diaphragm lifts and empties the lungs from the bottom. While this might seem opposed to "natural" breathing, try watching an infant breathing while he or she is sleeping. It is only as we grow older that most of us lose the capacity to draw optimum quantities of air into the lungs. While at first yogic breathing will require conscious effort, with practice it will become automatic and very comfortable.

Yogic breathing, unless otherwise specified, is always through the nose, not the mouth. In order to breathe properly the spine must be straight. This means the spine has to be carried like a column, with the shoulders back. This places the chest in an open position that does not constrict the lungs' capacity to expand. In the beginning you may feel you have to strain to fill the lungs, but soon your lung capacity will increase, given even a small amount of daily practice. Even more important than taking in larger quantities of air is the ability to exhale completely, emptying the lungs as much as possible. Asanas are designed to fill and empty areas of the lungs that our normal, more shallow breathing patterns do not reach.

After you are able to inhale/expand and exhale/contract, regulate your breath so that the incoming and outgoing breaths are balanced. In other words, try to make them the same approximate duration. You may mentally count to do this, but I find it preferable to develop an intuitive sense of timing. In order to develop this, in the initial stages I encourage my students to practice breathing as loudly as possible. The more air one takes in, the louder the noise. At first students react quite self-consciously to this exaggerated effort, but the purpose is to be able to direct one's hearing inward and simultaneously drown out or dampen external sounds with the repetitive sound of one's own breathing. An excellent mental practice to help with this is to imagine the incoming and outgoing breaths like waves on a shore, forever washing in and back out to sea, cycle upon cycle. When inner concentration develops one need not breathe as loudly, and in fact it becomes possible to take in very large quantities of air almost soundlessly.

There are a few basic breathing exercises that I practice. The first involves balancing the activity of the right and left nostrils. This is performed in order to balance and integrate the right and left sides of the brain. Using your right thumb, hold your right nostril shut and inhale through the left nostril. After drawing the air in, plug the left nostril as well, using the ring and little fingers. Hold your breath, then release the right nostril. Now repeat, inhaling through the right nostril. While various schools of yoga advise inhaling, holding, and exhaling to particular counts, I prefer people to set their own timing, with one stipulation: that the outgoing breath take at least as long to exhale as the incoming breath has taken on the inhale. Ideally, the exhalation should eventually become longer in duration than the inhalation. What is most important is to develop a pattern and stay with it during one session. I usually perform three rounds of this exercise (each round includes both left- and right-nostril breathing) as part of my morning yoga session.

The second exercise is *bastrika* or "breath of fire," an excellent way to clean out the lungs, increase oxygen intake, and energize consciousness. This exercise is almost like blowing your nose, so keep a handkerchief nearby. First, inhale using both nostrils. Then immediately contract your abdominal muscles and forcefully and rapidly expel the air from your lungs. Do this repeatedly, developing a pumping action at a medium to fast speed. While you should concentrate on breathing from your solar plexus, since it will be somewhat rapid your breathing may be more shallow than in other exercises. Again, the emphasis should be on the exhalation rather than on taking air in. After some time you might feel a bit light-headed, in which case you should slow down your breathing and inhale and exhale deeply and slowly three times. Do not overdo this exercise or you could actually pass out. In fact, you should always conclude bastrika with slow, deep breathing in order to stabilize your breath and return to normal consciousness before you try to stand up or move.

The final breathing exercise is called *kumbaka*. To practice kumbaka you must inhale, then hold that breath for as long as is comfortable. This should be practiced only after the inner and outer breaths are stabilized and equalized—once inhale/expand, exhale/contract becomes completely automatic. Kumbaka is an excellent way to deepen one's state of consciousness, whether practiced with eyes open or closed, for it offers a time-out from the ceaseless flux, a doorway into the inner realms. If it is used during meditation, one can very quickly reach a peaceful state. After many years of pranayama I sometimes find myself automatically practicing kumbaka in order to intensify my concentration while performing some task.

After kumbaka feels easy, start to leave a few seconds' gap not only between the inhalation and the exhalation but between the exhalation and the next inhalation as well. Then, in these few seconds of "fullness" or "emptiness," consciously direct all your attention inward and place it in the space that is created between breaths. Inhabit the peaceful stillness of that place. When you begin to breathe and move again, continue to hold the peacefulness. You will begin to inhabit what I call "the stillness in the midst of flow."

These breathing exercises should first be practiced in a seated position, preferably while sitting cross-legged on the floor. Once they become familiar, they should be practiced in conjunction with the asanas described later in this chapter.

Womb Yoga

Over the course of developing the asanas presented in this chapter, I used aspects of Indian dance movements as the basis of a general practice that would be useful to women of all ages. While many asanas are based on actual Indian dance movements or still poses, others are related to the dance in more indirect ways. Some were designed to prepare me for the dance, while still others were designed to counterbalance the effects of the movements of the dance (and other strains) on my lower back. In fact, a lengthy bout with lower back pain aggravated by the dance led me to consult the master hatha yogi B. K. S. Iyengar in Pune. When I asked him what I could do to correct my back pain, he knew exactly what to do—he commented that he had treated many of India's most famous dancers for the same problem. Then, in his characteristically brusque manner, he kindly, if not so subtly, obliged me with a suggestion. Grasping my shoulders from behind, he thrust his knee into my lower back and used it to push my entire pelvic area forward: "This is how the spine should be aligned," he said. His gesture, as abrupt as it seemed, told me what was most essential for me to know, and what was later confirmed by visits to chiropractors, physical therapists, and back specialists as well: that inordinate strain on the lower back needs to be counterbalanced by a realignment of the pelvis. The result is that now at least two-thirds of my warm-up exercises focus primarily on the lower back, and involve tilting the pelvis forward. Over time I have found that Indian dancers are not alone. Women of all ages experience problems with their lower backs, and many of my students have found relief from the asanas I developed to treat myself. Furthermore, I feel it is no coincidence that the area of weakness in the lower back corresponds to women's most vulnerable area, the region of the womb. For this reason I refer to the asanas that primarily benefit this area as "womb yoga."

By working this area one gains increasing control over the entire *manipura* chakra region, which is the center of will, vital to the well-being of not only women but men as well. After all, not only the womb but the vast majority of vital organs in both sexes are located in the same vicinity. However, for women this part of the body is especially important. In my yoga practice I concentrate heavily on the womb center for a reason. It seems to me that the center of will is the place where many of us on the planet need a lot of work. It is the pivotal center of our bodies, and the central point of balance in Indian dance. As the center of creativity, the womb is the source from which we all physically originate. Yet the womb as a symbol refers not only to the conception of human life but to creativity in general.

There is a continuum of energy between body, mind, and spirit. Womb yoga refers not only to the physical asanas used to strengthen this area of the body but to an awareness of the psychological factors that especially affect women's emotional and spiritual health. It begins by recognizing that the womb is one of our most problematic areas. After all, modern women have struggled hard to escape the "anatomy is destiny" status of being reduced to our reproductive role. Since the advent of the birth control pill women's sexuality no longer inevitably results in pregnancy, so we are free to express our sexuality for pleasure rather than only for the purpose of reproduction. As a result, for the first time in history our collective eroticism overflows the bounds of family and can express itself as a larger sense of relatedness to society and the world. This manifests not only in sexual freedom—which can easily turn into its own kind of slavery—but, more positively, in both individual and collective social actions that seek nothing less than the transformation of the planet. Around the world women's development and social activist movements are no less a feature of the political landscape than the burgeoning global economic market.

Yet, as we move forward into the light, there is a shadow cast by this rapid feminine evolutionary development. It's name is fear. We carry it within us, an unconscious fear of being forced or even seduced back into what many of us view as a kind of slavery to the womb. This fear often becomes internalized, projected onto our own bodies in the form of guilt or anger, and becomes localized in the region of the womb. At the very least we are culturally predisposed to view our wombs as superfluous; at worst, as an enemy to our higher selves. For birth control we block or circumvent the womb's natural functions; then, when we actually want to conceive, many of us are unable to do so. Finally, throughout our lives we are programmed to rely on gynecologists to monitor our wombs, as if they were danger zones. I cannot help but suspect that the effects of this scenario might have something to do with the high rate of reproductive and hormonal disorders among women of all ages in our culture.

Womb yoga offers a way to consciously face these problems and to reestablish our relationship with our bodies and our psyches beginning at the center, by starting where it all began, our point of origin. I encourage my students to breathe life, consciousness, and energy into the areas of the second and third chakras. By working the muscles of the lower abdominal and vaginal regions during inhalation/expansion and exhalation/contraction, and simultaneously visualizing the sending of healing light into the area, the entire womb area is infused with new life and energy.

To understand the larger dimensions of our own power we must move beyond a primarily biological understanding of creativity. We must begin to positively recognize the womb as a powerful feeling center in women, from which place we can begin to heal not only ourselves but the world. It is not only through our hearts that we experience our connections to family, lovers, and the world at large. Closer to the earth than the heart, the type of feelings we experience in our wombs are more instinctual, harder to put into words but no less intensely felt or necessary for the survival of our whole being. Any woman who has carried life in her womb or who has given birth knows of the powerful nature of these feelings. Birth contractions are like an earthquake that rocks us to the core of our being; similarly, intense sexual desire spreads a kind of heat throughout the womb area, while elemental fear is often felt there like a sharp blow. Pain or emotional sensitivity around the time of menstruation is explained away in chemical terms, the result of increased hormone production, but it is also deeply symbolic of women's connection to the earth. Just as the tides respond to the moon, so do the "tides" within women.

I have myself experienced the kind of sorrow that is felt like a dull blow in the area of the womb. If I am hurt I find myself automatically placing my hands over my heart, as if to protect it. But if I am very deeply disturbed, often over something that is happening in the larger world—for example, reading in the newspaper or hearing on the radio about some great tragedy, injustice, or suffering—I sometimes double over in physical pain. There have been times when I have felt so heavy I feel as if I am carrying the entire planet inside my womb. These feelings should not be denied or repressed. In such times I curl into a fetal position and meditate, offering healing prayers for the world. Like the heart, the womb is a place in us where fear and anger can become transformed into compassion, where our individual emotions can and do feed into the collective spiritual climate of the planet.

The Chakras

While the womb center is a place from which to begin to heal our bodies, we must also work with a larger picture of the body. Because our goal is total integration, before we begin the actual asanas it is important to develop a basic understanding of each of the chakras: their physical, emotional, and spiritual aspects. In the asanas that follow I will refer to various chakras for visualization purposes.

The first and lowest chakra is the *muladhara,* located between the anus and the sexual organs. The muladhara relates to the physical foundations of life—the eliminatory function and the immune system, as well as the bones, the overall structure on which our bodies are built. The second chakra is the *svadisthana,* located in women in the *yoni,* the region of the vulva and vagina, and in men at the base of the penis. This is the center that governs the sexual and reproductive organs, as well as the lower intestines and the bladder. The muladhara and svadisthana are located so close to each other that disorders in one region are almost sure to affect the other. The third chakra is called the *manipura,* the center of the will. It governs the organs of digestion and the vast majority of physical functions that relate to the quality of our life. Located just below the navel, it is the center of the "lower" emotions like fear and envy, emotions related to one's survival in the world. The fourth chakra is the heart center, the *anahata.* Physically related to the circulatory and respiratory systems, it is also the center of the primary emotions: love and sorrow. The heart chakra mediates the "lower" and "higher" functions of the personality, the physical with the psychic, the body with the head. The fifth chakra is located at the throat and is called the *vishuddha* chakra. This is the center of verbal communication, governing the vocal chords and the windpipe, but the mouth is also the home of taste, the starting point of the digestive tract. The fifth chakra is the primary site of conscious self-representation, as so many of our thoughts get transformed into speech.

The two higher chakras are located in the head, beginning with the *ajna,* located in the forehead between the eyebrows. This is the "third eye" of Hindu and Buddhist traditions, and is related to the pineal or the "master gland," located in the center of the brain, which governs all the other glandular systems in the body. The ajna chakra is also related to the eyes and corresponds to the physical sensation of sight. Finally the last and highest chakra in the body is the *sahasrara,* or "thousand-petaled lotus." This is the seat of consciousness, located in the top of the skull. This center governs the higher functions of the brain, and out of this region emerges one's "higher" conceptualizations of self and world.

In understanding the chakra system as a whole, it is interesting to note the hierarchy that emerges. Generally speaking, within the body "higher" and "lower" chakras respectively translate into "subtle" and "gross." The lowest chakras are concerned with the raw physicality of the earth—the production of wastes from digestion, in the case of the first chakra, and the production of human bodies in the second chakra. Conversely, the highest chakras are concerned with the production of that which is more subtle: speech, thought, and conceptualization. And yet to so completely divide the domain and function of the chakras is also inaccurate, as what is even more important than any of the chakras' separate functions is their total integration. In reality, each chakra's particular function in working for the entire organism is totally dependent upon all the others. Each chakra may be understood to encompass and reflect, on another level, the one that comes before it. For example the third, manipura, chakra, the center of creative will in human beings, is a more subtle reflection of the natural creative or life-giving properties of the second chakra, which rules human sexuality and reproduction.

As yoginis we must conceive of a new liberation, one that does not seek a simplistic transcendence but rather a complex integration. Realizing the union of body, soul, and spirit, of the male and female within, we must seed our own wombs, our creative centers, with our dreams and visions, in order to give birth to ourselves and a new conception of life. I know that I am not alone in this conviction. Countless women throughout the planet are undergoing "labor" on all levels, in the hopes of bringing a new consciousness and physical reality into being. By using yogic techniques that integrate the emotional and physical with the spiritual, women, and men who have the courage to resonate with their own feminine power, can strengthen themselves not only to resist the negativity of these tumultuous times but to positively influence the direction of life on earth.

Beginning the Asanas

In the following section I offer my own individualized yoga program to others who may be interested in incorporating aspects of Indian classical dance into their yoga practice. I have grouped the yogini asanas according to the basic stance of each—according to whether they are performed standing, seated, or on the ground. In anticipation of the last chapter of this book, "Yoga of the Elements," I also relate each of these groups to one of the *panchabhuta* or five elements: earth, water, fire, air, and space. Either in the introduction to the asana or in the "key" section that follows each, I offer suggestions regarding which chakra to activate; this is achieved by placing one's awareness at that center. I also offer a "benefits" comment on each posture, so that readers can immediately identify asanas for particular areas of the body that need work.

Before we go any farther I must remind readers of an important point that I continually stress in my yoga classes. You must discover for yourself which yogini asanas are most appropriate given your body structure, daily patterns of movement, and ultimate purpose for practicing yoga. In other words, regardless of its traditional framework, yoga need not be viewed as a set number of predetermined positions into which one tries to force one's body. Rather, it is a process of discovering your inner awareness and sensitivity, and bringing that into balance with outer form. As I have repeatedly stated, what is most important in practicing yoga is the consciousness one brings to it. Only by tuning in at this level will you become aware of the subtle flow of energy that is always available to you.

To practice these asanas I recommend that you first concentrate on the physical positions and breathing. When you try the various positions there are bound to be some to which your body will not conform. Do not be concerned. Instead, approximate the position and concentrate on the breathing. From the outset, try to practice the asanas as best you can in conjunction with the proper breathing pattern: inhale/expand, exhale/contract. When you reach the limits of any given movement do not try to force yourself into a position; instead, relax and breathe into it further, concentrating inwardly on the sensation you are experiencing. Learn to distinguish between discomfort and actual pain. If you feel pain, relax further, breathe, and if necessary retreat from the "edge," the limit of your physical ability. You will find that over a period of time this limit will also move as your flexibility increases. Once you have reached the edge *without* pain (though there may be discomfort), hold the position and imagine that you have attained the ideal form, all the while practicing conscious and relaxed breathing.

When you are satisfied with the physical position or movement and can do it almost automatically, begin to draw your attention inward, away from the external form, and feel the flow of energy that travels with the breath. Scanning your body internally, you may become aware of areas where there are "knots" or tight spots, areas of tenseness or discomfort. Visualize and direct relaxing, healing breath and energy to those areas.

In order to coordinate the movement, breathing, and visualization in these asanas I have found that, at least initially, it is better to perform the asanas as slowly as possible. In order to establish a slow, flowing pace, try practicing to meditative music, either Indian or western, and synchronize your breathing with the tempo. Repetitive, hypnotic music will automatically draw your attention inward. If you are particularly distracted and need to make an extra effort to concentrate, perform the asanas with your eyes closed. I prefer to do yoga with eyes open, because I enjoy looking at the world and at parts of my own body from the different angles produced by the asanas. You might try that after you become more established in your practice. As you learn to focus on the inner sensations that arise from various organs and limbs you will be able to give yourself your own physical and mental "checkup." I use yoga to "ground" myself in the here and now in this way, after a night of dreams, before beginning my daily work.

Finally, when practicing yoga remember to create a good mood for yourself. Just as when I enter the stage for a dance performance, no matter how tense I feel I begin with a smile on my face. When doing yoga, as well, if you put a gentle expression on your face it is not long before *santa rasa,* the peaceful emotion, arises from within and transforms your yoga session into a genuine pleasure. Over time, your entire perception of what it means to be physically fit will change. Your standards of fitness will increase along with your awareness, and your practice of yoga will be transformed from an exercise to an art. Asanas will naturally flow into each other. Soon you will find yourself immersed in the dance of yoga.

Sixty-Four Yogini Asanas

Standing Asanas
(Element: Space)

I usually begin my practice with a few standing asanas in order to establish a sense of my body in the midst of space. As many as possible involve facing forward, backward, to the right and left, and even up and down, to help me to fully locate myself in the here and now of three-dimensional space. While the following asanas seem simple, they are extremely important in balancing the body—creating a symmetry between the right and left halves of the body. By straightening and stretching the spine, they are also the first steps toward better overall posture.

I also use these asanas to establish my yoga practice in relation to Indian classical dance, which begins from a basic standing posture. Do this by locating your body's pivotal center at the third chakra, just below the navel. Placing your awareness at that center, settle down and let yourself fully inhabit your body. In this way you create a solid standing foundation from which to move outward. Imagine the movements that follow to be the movements of a dance.

The following mudras (or *hastas,* as they are referred to in dance texts) will be used throughout this section, in conjunction with various asanas. These mudras are common in Indian classical dance; in abstract dance they have a decorative function, whereas in representational dance they carry specific meanings—they either symbolize a concept or portray some kind of activity. Based on the classical dance texts there are twenty-eight single hand gestures and twenty-three double hand gestures, constituting a sign language that even today is understood by educated audiences in India.

To learn dance is to learn this language, which transcends the written and spoken word. It directly conveys a variety of meanings—mental, emotional, and spiritual. As well, similar to their use in religious ritual, hand gestures "seal in" the energy that flows through the dancer's limbs, either recirculating that energy back into the performer's body or directing it outward toward the audience in a highly focused manner.

Pataka mudra, "the flag," is formed by joining and extending all your fingers straight up, creating

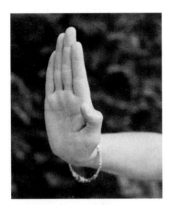

Pataka mudra,
"the flag"

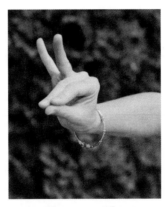

Hamsasya mudra,
"the swan's beak"

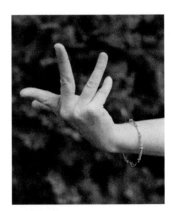

Alapadma mudra,
"the full lotus"

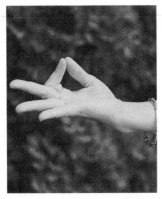

Arala mudra,
"the bend"

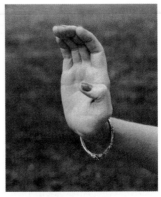

Sarpasirsa mudra,
"the cobra's hood"

a flat surface of your palm. *Hamsasya* mudra, "the swan's beak," is formed by bringing your first two fingers to meet your thumb while extending and spreading the other two fingers (ring and little fingers) straight upward. *Alapadma,* "the full lotus," is formed by spreading all the fingers wide open, with the thumb pointed down toward the earth, the index finger extending outward in line with the forearm, the little finger pointing back toward the forearm, and the remaining fingers spread as far apart as possible like a fan. *Arala,* "the bend," is created with a flat palm, when you bend your index finger and join it to your thumb. This hand position increases concentration by completing the energy circuit, and hence "recirculates" energy back into the body. Finally, *sarpasirsa,* "the cobra's hood," is created by performing the pataka or flat-palm mudra, and then bending the tips of your first three fingers forward. You can join two sarpasirsa mudras by linking thumbs while holding both hands in this position.

When practicing these asanas, remember that, as a species, human beings are the only animals who are able to stand in an upright posture, with the spine perpendicular to the earth. This ability to defy gravity represents the beginning of humankind's transcendence and journey toward that unknown called Spirit. Extend yourself upward and claim your rightful place in the cosmos!

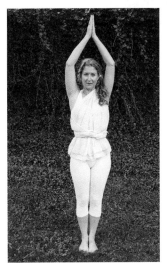

Figure 1.1

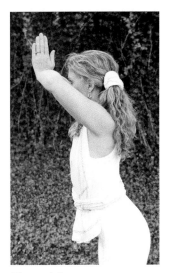

Figure 1.2

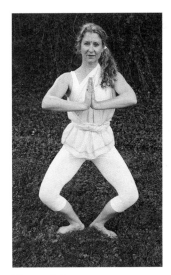

Figure 1.3

Vertical Stretch

Begin in a simple standing posture, feet together. Place your hands above your head, palms together, flattening the curvature of your spine by tilting your pelvis forward (fig. 1.1). Maintaining this position, inhale and exhale three times while keeping your spine straight and fully stretched. Inhale for the fourth time. On the exhale, lower your joined palms in front of your forehead, shifting your upper body slightly forward (fig. 1.2). Maintaining this position, inhale and exhale three times.

On the fourth exhalation lower your joined palms in front of your heart (fig. 1.3). Turn your feet out and bend your knees, spreading them out to the

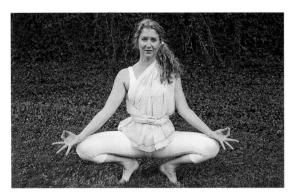

Figure 1.4

side. Hold your pelvis slightly forward; do not allow your lower back to bow inward. Maintaining this position, inhale and exhale three times.

On the fourth exhalation, fully spread your knees out to the side and lower your body until you are balancing on your ankles, your hands resting on your knees (fig. 1.4). Keep your back straight. Hold this position and breathe deeply three times.

To complete the asana reverse the process, returning to a standing position by moving upward through the previous asanas. Remember to move on the exhalations, not the inhalations.

Key: Control your abdominal muscles. Concentrate your attention on and breathe from the manipura chakra, the womb center located a few inches below your navel. Expand your abdominal muscles on the inhalation and contract them on every exhalation.

Benefits: This asana stretches the spine and leg muscles, and tones the abdomen.

Forward Bend

Beginning again in a simple standing posture, feet together, place your hands above your head with palms together. Then flatten the curvature of your spine by tilting your pelvis forward (fig. 2.1). Inhale and exhale while holding your spine in this flattened

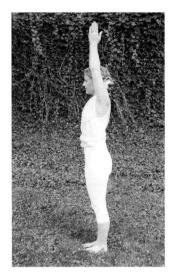

Figure 2.1

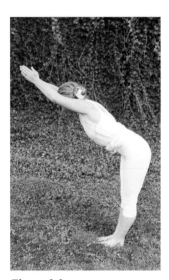

Figure 2.2

position. Inhale a second time. On the exhale, while still keeping the spine flat, contract your abdominal muscles and lean forward approximately forty-five degrees (fig. 2.2). Maintaining that position, inhale, expanding your abdominal muscles and keeping your arms fully extended above your head. On the exhale, lean forward so that your upper body is perpendicular to your lower body (fig. 2.3).

Inhale once more and bring your arms around to the back, interlacing your fingers (fig. 2.4). On the exhalation, lift your arms while dropping your

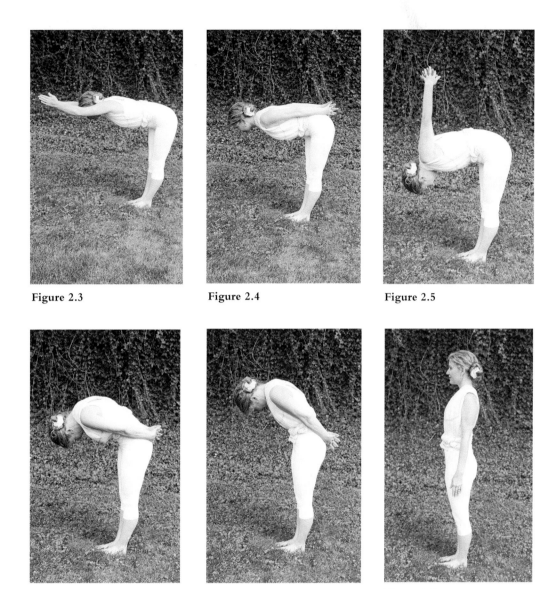

Figure 2.3

Figure 2.4

Figure 2.5

Figure 2.6

Figure 2.7

Figure 2.8

head forward and looking at the ground. Keep your back parallel to the ground (fig. 2.5).

On an inhale, slowly roll your spine upward and return to the original standing position (figs. 2.6 and 2.7). With your hands still linked behind your back, inhale, then exhale, bringing your arms down to your sides (fig. 2.8).

Key: In leaning forward, keep your spine fully extended and your balance point as far forward as possible.

Benefits: This asana strengthens the abdomen and lower back muscles.

※

The following asana is taken from the basic stance of Indian classical dance, one in which the arms are extended out to the side at shoulder level. In dance class we are required to stand in this pose while reciting the appropriate verses of the Natya Sastra *that describe the various mudras, or hand positions, used in the dance, and to execute them one by one. The following exercise strengthens the muscles of the arm by consciously stretching them into a fully extended position while simultaneously rotating them from back to front.*

Horizontal Arm Stretch

Begin by standing with your feet about six inches apart, your knees slightly bent and your pelvis tipped slightly forward (fig. 3.1). Find a solid footing. Extend your arms out to your sides, level with your shoulders, your palms facing down (fig. 3.2). Keeping your arms fully extended, on an inhale rotate your arms backward until your palms face up and back. Let your head and neck follow the rotation until you are looking skyward (fig. 3.3). Keep your lower back stationary; stretch only your upper back and neck muscles. To "seal" or lock in energy, use the alapadma mudra, consciously stretching your fingers.

On the exhale, rotate your arms fully forward until the entire underside of your arm faces upward. Let your head follow, until your chin is

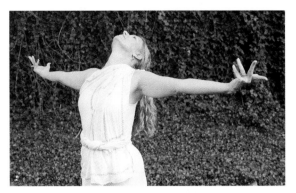

Figure 3.3

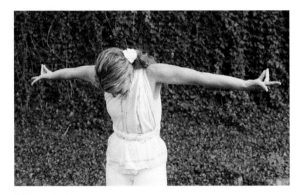

Figure 3.4

resting on your chest (fig. 3.4). During this last movement, slowly transform your hand positions from alapadma mudra into hamsasya mudra.

Repeat the sequence from upward rotation to downward rotation for at least three rounds. Complete the asana by coming to the original standing position, facing front. Lower arms slowly to your sides.

Key: Be sure to hold the basic stance so that your back moves as little as possible. Focus on opening the chest region by placing your concentration at the anahata chakra, located in the region of the heart, while continuing to work your abdominal muscles on the inhalation and exhalation.

Benefits: This asana stretches your upper back and neck muscles and releases tension from the shoulder area.

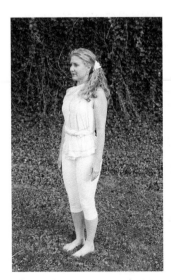 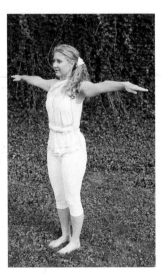

Figure 3.1   **Figure 3.2**

The following two asanas are based on dance sculptures carved on the outside of Indian temples like those at Konarak, where languorous women stand with one arm raised above their heads, one knee lifted out to the side. Modifying this image into a yogini asana, I have stylized it into a meditation on balance and relaxed poise: while rotating my arms I coordinate the rate of my incoming and outgoing breath, and concentrate on keeping them in perfect synchronization. For this asana, imagine energy flowing between the heart (anahata chakra) and the lower two chakras, the muladhara and svadisthana, located at the lowest point of the torso, in the region of the anus and yoni (vulva and vagina). When you find yourself losing balance, move the energy to the lower regions in order to draw stability from the earth.

Vertical Arm Stretch

Begin by standing with your feet slightly apart, your knees bent slightly and your pelvis tipped slightly forward. With your hands in front of your chest, place your left hand in pataka mudra, palm down, on top of your right hand, palm up (fig. 4.1). On the inhale, pass your left arm in front of your body, raising it above your head, your left palm facing skyward; simultaneously extend your right arm downward, turning at the wrist so that your right palm faces the earth (fig. 4.2).

Both hands rotate in this movement, the upward-moving hand rotating up and out from your body while the downward-moving hand turns inward toward your body, then down. Both hands should end up at right angles to your arms. Extend your arms fully without tipping the horizontal line of your shoulders.

On the exhale, reverse the movement and bring your hands back in front of your chest, with the left palm returning to rest on top of the right.

Now switch hands so that the right hand is resting on the left (fig. 4.3). Repeat the same movements on the opposite side (fig. 4.4).

Alternating sides, repeat the entire sequence four times.

Now coordinate the movements of your arms with leg lifts. After repeating the Vertical Arm

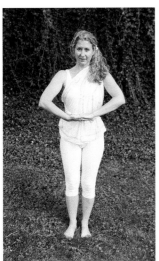

Figure 4.1

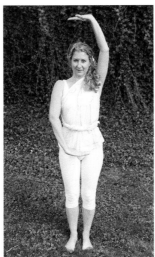

Figure 4.2

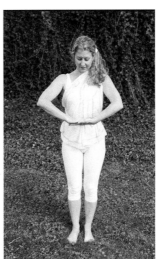

Figure 4.3

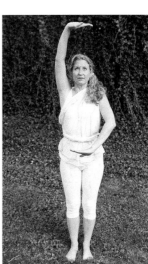

Figure 4.4

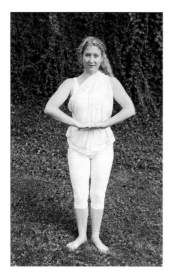
Figure 4.5

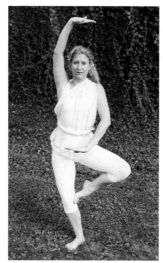
Figure 4.6

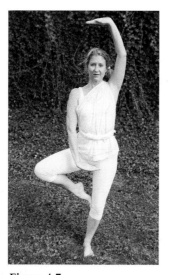
Figure 4.7

Exhale and come back to the starting position.

Switch sides, this time lifting the right leg as you raise your left arm (fig. 4.7). Alternate sides, repeating the entire sequence three times.

Key: To create a graceful flow, rotate your hands at the beginning of the movement. Regulate your breath with the flow of the movements. Try to keep your back straight and your pelvis slightly forward, despite your raised leg.

Benefits: This asana tones your arm muscles and balances the right and left sides of your body. Adding the leg raises will increase the mobility of your hips and strengthen the lateral muscles of your thighs.

For this asana, extend the energy flow farther upward to the region of the vishuddha chakra (in the throat area). At the same time remain grounded by the solid stance of the unlocked knee position, and by keeping a part of your awareness in the lowest chakra.

Extended Arm Rotation

Begin by standing with your feet six inches apart, your knees slightly bent and your pelvis tipped slightly forward. With your hands in pataka mudra, extend your arms out to the side, as in the Horizontal Arm Stretch (fig. 5.1).

On the inhale, extend your right arm upward, palm up, and your left arm straight down behind your lower back, palm down. Once fully extended, your hands should be at right angles to your arms (fig. 5.2). On the exhale, bend your elbows and extend your arms until your fingers overlap behind your back (fig. 5.3). Inhale and exhale, holding this position.

Stretch four times, return to standing with your feet slightly apart and turned forty-five degrees out to the side (fig. 4.5). This time let your right hand rest in pataka mudra, palm down, on top of your left hand. As you raise your right hand over your head, bend your left knee and lift it up and out to the side, keeping your raised foot close to your leg (fig. 4.6). Keep your toe pointed and bring your raised foot to knee level or above.

Hold this position through one breathing cycle.

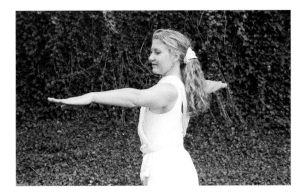

Figure 5.1

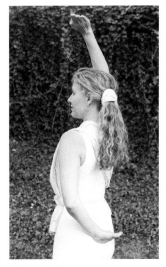

Figure 5.2

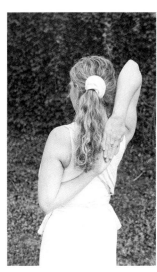

Figure 5.3

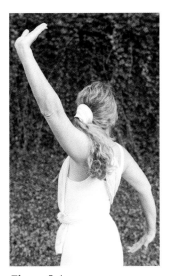

Figure 5.4

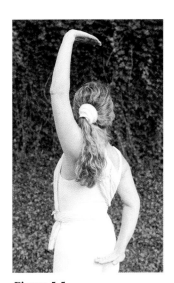

Figure 5.5

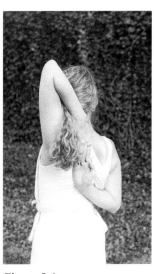

Figure 5.6

On the next inhalation, stretch your arms out vertically behind your back. Extend them fully, then rotate them up and around (fig. 5.4), until your left hand is over your head, palm up, and your right hand is behind your back, palm down (fig. 5.5). On the exhale, bend your elbows and move your arms until your fingers overlap (fig. 5.6). Hold this position for one breath cycle, then extend your arms vertically and change sides once again.

Repeat this asana three times, alternating sides.

Key: Once you straighten your arms, keep them fully extended until you reach the next position. Be sure to keep your back straight; a swayback position makes it easier to overlap your fingers, but such a position will not benefit your lower back.

Benefits: This asana results in an extended range of movement in the shoulders, and develops the inner muscles of your upper arms.

> *The following asana allows you to practice consciously visualizing the position of your body from the outside. Three different poses are created by bending the knees, adjusting the spine, and shifting the weight. Visualize your body as it would appear from a sideways perspective.*

Extended Standing Stretch

To begin, stand with your legs together, your hands at your sides (fig. 6.1). Inhale and raise your arms over your head, palms together, fingers interlocked, forefingers extended (fig. 6.2).

On the exhale, step forward on your right leg so that your right foot is about twelve inches in front of the left, your toes pointing forward, and tilt your pelvis slightly forward so that your back feels perfectly straight. Keep your legs straight at the knees. At the same time, lower your arms until they are extended straight out ahead of you (fig. 6.3). Inhale and raise your arms upward once more, stretching your spine and pulling upward (fig. 6.4).

On the next exhalation, bend your right knee and lean forward so that your right knee is over the toes of your right foot. Bend your elbows and stretch your arms back over your head (fig. 6.5). Tilting your head back, look up. Exhale and inhale. On the next exhalation return to a straight standing position, your arms over your head (fig. 6.6). Inhale in place.

Now exhale and, contracting your abdomen, bend your left knee and slightly tilt your pelvis forward while you lean your hips back. Your thighs and knees will be lined up evenly. Extend your arms straight out in front of you, palms together (fig. 6.7). Inhale in place. On exhale, return to a straight standing position (fig. 6.8).

Repeat the asana series, bringing the left foot forward.

Key: Concentrate on breathing from the manipura chakra (solar plexus area). When leaning back, contract your abdominal muscles completely, pulling your navel back toward your spine.

Benefits: This is an excellent stretch for your leg and arm muscles, as well as your lower spine.

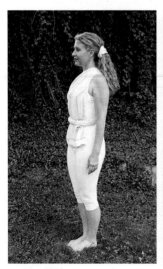
Figure 6.1

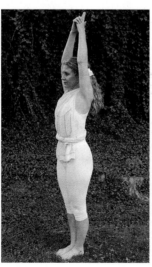
Figure 6.2

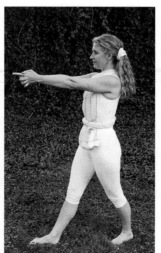
Figure 6.3

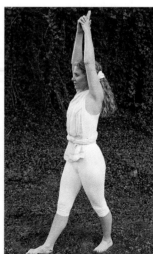
Figure 6.4

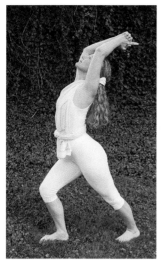 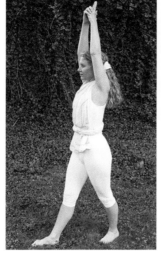 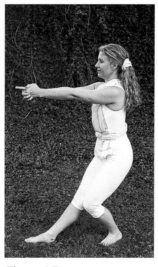 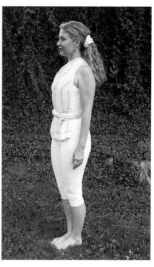

Figure 6.5   Figure 6.6   Figure 6.7   Figure 6.8

The following two asanas are preparation for the basic position of South Indian classical dance, which involves a half-squat position, knees turned out to the sides. These exercises bring you close to the earth while still in a standing position. Concentrate your awareness in the lowest two chakras (muladhara and svadisthana) below the base of the spine and, when in the fully seated position, consciously draw energy from the earth.

The Squat

Begin by squatting on the ground, your feet flat on the ground and slightly apart, your toes turned out to the side. Resting your forearms on the ground in front of you, focus your vision just past your hands (fig 7.1). Try to keep your back as straight as possible in this position in order to stretch the lower back. Inhale and exhale in place.

On the exhale, flatten your back farther and sit up so that only your hands and feet are resting on the ground (fig. 7.2). Inhale and exhale in place. On exhale, lower your head and slowly raise your body up, still keeping your feet flat on the ground (figs. 7.3 and 7.4). Hold this position and breathe.

On an exhale, straighten your legs and drop your head as close to your knees as possible, hands and feet flat on the ground (fig. 7.4). Hold this position and breathe.

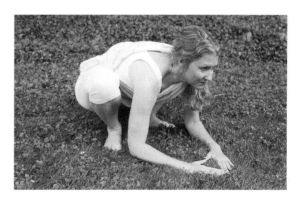

Figure 7.1

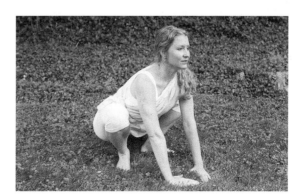

Figure 7.2

THE DANCE OF YOGA ※ 79

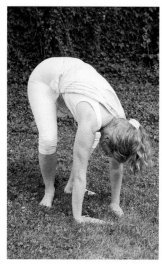
Figure 7.3

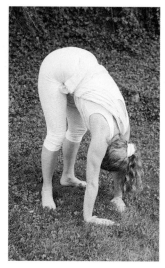
Figure 7.4

Benefits: This asana draws energy to the lower extremities. At the same time it works the muscles of both your upper and lower back and stretches the muscles along the back of your legs. The inverted (head-down) position draws blood to the face and increases circulation in the brain.

The Extended Squat

Stand with your feet apart, toes pointed outward about forty-five degrees, palms joined in front of your chest and hips tilted slightly forward (fig. 8.1). Inhale and exhale in this position. On your next inhale, raise up on your toes and extend your arms upward at forty-five-degree angles, your hands in alapadma mudra (fig. 8.2).

On exhale, bend your knees and lower yourself to a squatting position, lowering your arms down slowly until they rest on your knees, your hands in arala mudra (fig. 8.3). Hold this position and inhale, exhale, and inhale again. On exhale, stand up slowly, returning to the starting position (fig. 8.4).

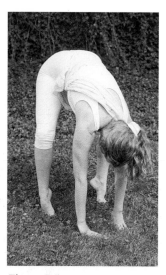
Figure 7.5

Finally, on an exhale extend your ankles so that you are standing on your tiptoes, knees spread out to the side (fig. 7.5). In time with your breathing, alternately bend and straighten your feet and legs. To finish, slowly roll up to a standing position.

Key: To feel the energy in the lower chakras, expand and contract your anal, vaginal, and abdominal muscles with the breathing, even while bent over.

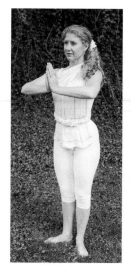
Figure 8.1

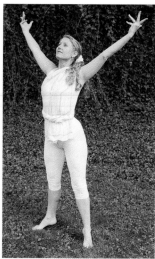
Figure 8.2

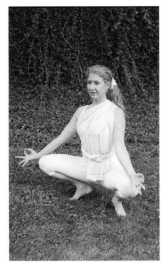
Figure 8.3

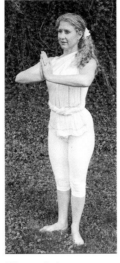
Figure 8.4

Key: Notice that in this squatting position your legs are much farther apart than in the preceding asana.

Benefits: This asana will thoroughly stretch and strengthen your leg muscles, especially your thighs. This asana is not recommended for overweight persons or those with weak knees.

Asanas on the Earth
(Element: Earth)

These asanas are extremely grounding and sensual. They place the body in full contact with Mother Earth. Sometimes giving in to her embrace, at other times feeling the full force of her downward pull as we lift ourselves away from her, we come to intimately know ourselves as both a part of Earth and yet distinct from her. Through the weight of our own bodies we develop strength; through concentrated effort we develop grace in the face of gravity.

༄

The following "Bridge" asana series is most effective for locating and energizing the manipura chakra, the womb center of the will. By breathing into this area and visualizing the flow of energy in the form of light, you will actually feel the blood flowing into the area of the vital organs and the lower back.

Raising the Bridge

Lie flat on the ground, arms at your sides. On exhalation, contract your abdominal muscles and tilt your pelvis slightly upward, flattening your spine until it is in contact with the earth from neck to tailbone (fig. 9.1). Inhale and expand your belly as much as possible, being careful not to move your spine.

Lower your chin slightly to expose your spine at the neck. Now exhale and contract your belly,

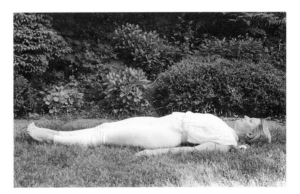
Figure 9.1

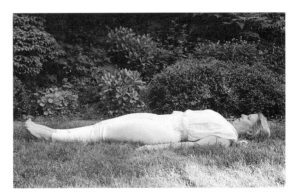
Figure 9.2

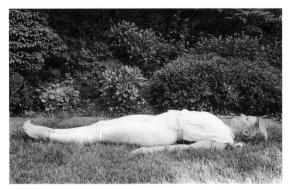

Figure 9.3

at the same time trying to relax your limbs as much as possible (fig. 9.2). The only muscles that should be tense are those of the abdomen and lower back.

Continuing to hold your spine against the ground, breathe deeply for four rounds. To finish, completely relax your whole body, including your spine, and breathe for another four rounds (fig. 9.3).

Key: The benefit of this asana is all in the breathing. Focus your full awareness on the manipura chakra, a few inches below the navel, and inhale/expand, exhale/contract.

Benefits: This asana strengthens your lower back and the muscles of the abdominal region.

Raising the Bridge II

Lie on your back, bending your knees until your spine is flat against the ground (fig. 10.1). Keeping your neck and shoulders on the ground, inhale and raise your hips slowly, until your back creates a flat plane from your chest to your knees (fig. 10.2). Expand your abdominal muscles on inhalation as much as possible. Hold this position and exhale, fully contracting your abdominal muscles.

Perform three cycles of breathing in this position. On the fourth exhalation, lower your spine halfway to the ground (fig. 10.3). Hold this position and repeat three more cycles of breathing. On the fourth exhalation, lower your spine so it is just resting on the ground, your hips and pelvis still tilted upward (fig. 10.4).

Perform three breathing cycles. On the fourth inhalation, once again raise your hips to their maximum height, expanding your abdominal muscles (fig. 10.5). Hold your breath for a count of four,

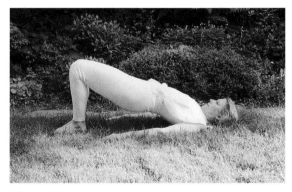

Figure 10.2

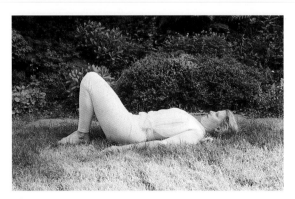

Figure 10.1

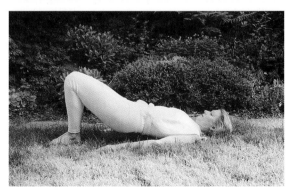

Figure 10.3

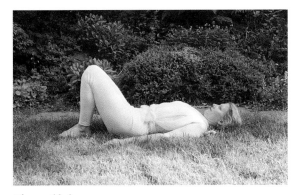

Figure 10.4

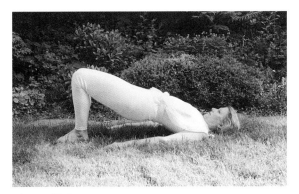

Figure 10.5

Exhale, slowly stretching your straight leg up, outward, and down until it reaches the ground, raising your hips as your leg moves downward (figs. 11.4, 11.5, and 11.6). You have created a one-legged bridge. If necessary, use pressure on your upper arms at each side to stabilize yourself. Hold this position and inhale.

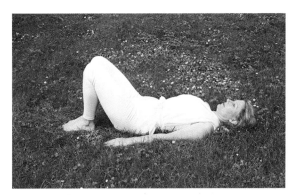

Figure 11.1

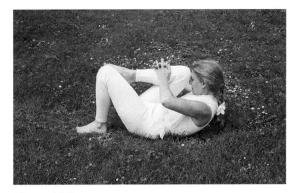

Figure 11.2

then exhale, lowering your back to the ground but still maintaining an upward-tilted pelvis. Your entire spine should be in contact with the earth.

Repeat this asana three times through.

Key: This sequence should be performed as slowly as possible, coordinating the rate of your deep breathing with slow and deliberate movements.

Benefits: This asana further strengthens your lower back and the muscles of the abdominal region.

Raising the Bridge III

Lie on your back with bent knees, your spine flat on the ground. Inhale in this position (fig. 11.1). Exhale, drawing your right knee up and lifting your head and shoulders until your knee touches your forehead (fig. 11.2). Inhale and straighten your right leg (fig. 11.3).

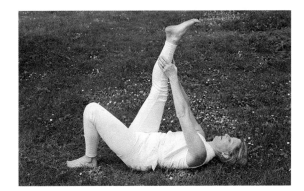

Figure 11.3

THE DANCE OF YOGA ❦ 83

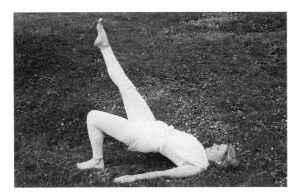

Figure 11.4

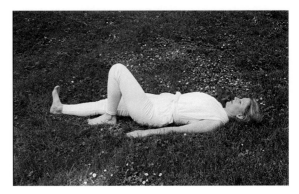

Figure 11.7

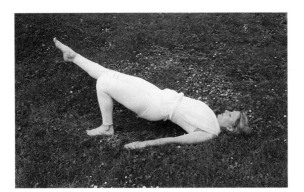

Figure 11.5

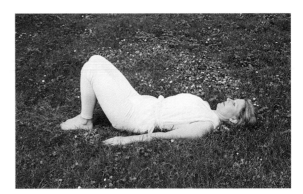

Figure 11.8

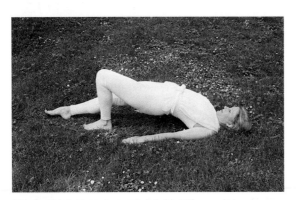

Figure 11.6

Exhale and slowly lower your spine back to the ground; finish by flexing the ankle of the lowered leg (fig. 11.7).

Inhale slowly and bring your right leg to a bent-knee position (fig. 11.8). Perform the asana raising the left leg.

Repeat three times each side.

Key: Stretch your leg out as far as possible, point-ing your toe until your foot reaches the ground.

Benefits: This asana stretches the leg muscles as it further strengthens the lower back.

Raising the Bridge IV

Lie on your back, your spine flat on the ground, your knees bent so that your feet are close to your buttocks (fig. 12.1). Inhale deeply.

On exhale, spread your knees apart as wide as possible so that your legs come to rest on the ground, the soles of your feet joined together (fig. 12.2). In this position, try to relax your leg muscles as much as possible. Inhale/expand and exhale/contract, working your abdominal muscles as you breathe.

On the second exhalation, lift your hips off the ground and raise them as high as is comfortable (fig. 12.3). This will bring your knees closer

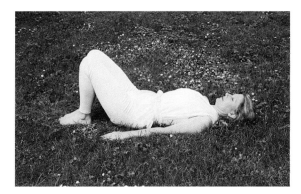

Figure 12.1

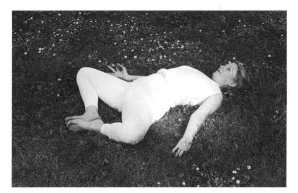

Figure 12.2

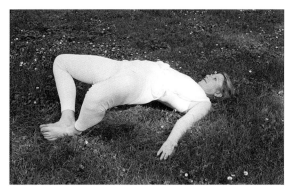

Figure 12.3

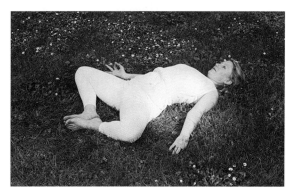

Figure 12.4

together, but your knees should still be kept as far apart as is possible. Hold this position and breathe, inhaling and exhaling three times.

On the fourth exhalation, slowly lower your back to the ground (fig. 12.4). Flatten your spine against the earth and breathe deeply.

Key: To effectively perform this asana you must be able to bear your weight on the sides of your feet.

If this causes discomfort, do not hold the raised position for longer than ten or fifteen seconds.

Benefits: This asana stretches your thigh muscles as it strengthens the lower back.

Raising the Side Bridge

Lie on your back with your spine on the ground, knees out to the side and the soles of your feet together (fig. 13.1). Your arms are at your sides. Inhale and exhale for two cycles. On the second exhalation, raise your right knee so that your right foot is flat on the ground while your left knee remains on the ground (fig. 13.2).

On the inhale, lift your pelvis off the ground as much as possible (fig. 13.3). (This may not be too far, possibly only a few inches.) Lower your pelvis on exhale.

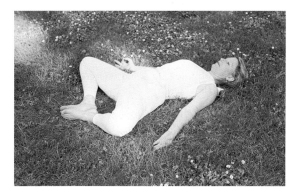

Figure 13.1

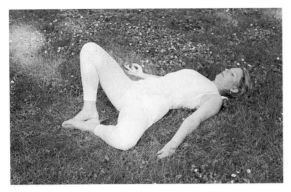

Figure 13.2

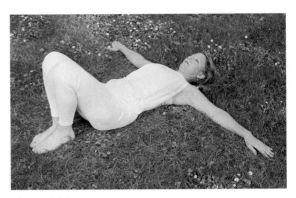

Figure 14.1

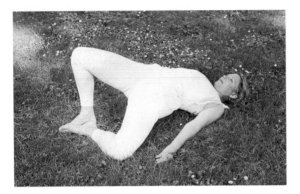

Figure 13.3

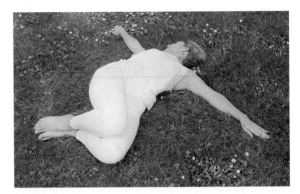

Figure 14.2

Repeat three times on each side. On the final exhalation, return to the starting position.

Key: Concentrate on breathing into the abdominal region, the womb center, where pressure is exerted when you raise your hips slightly off the ground. There is no need to hold this position for more than one round of breathing.

Benefits: This exercise massages your internal organs while further strengthening the lower back muscles.

Lowering the Bridge I

Lie with your spine flat against the earth, your pelvis tipped slightly upward. Bend your knees so that your feet are close to your buttocks; feet and ankles are together (fig. 14.1). Extend your arms straight out to the side. Inhale in place.

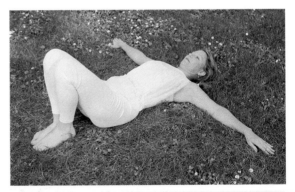

Figure 14.3

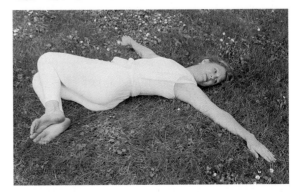

Figure 14.4

On the exhale, slowly lower your bent knees to the left until they rest on the ground, while simultaneously turning your head fully to the right (fig. 14.2). Look at your right hand. Inhale and exhale in place.

On the next inhale, raise your knees to the starting position while you turn your head back to center (fig. 14.3). On exhale, lower your knees to the right and look left (fig. 14.4).

Repeat this sequence three times on each side.

Key: Perform the entire sequence slowly and deliberately, feeling the stretch across your body and breathing into it.

Benefits: This asana stretches your entire torso and firms your waist.

Lowering the Bridge II

Once again, lie with your spine flat against the earth. Bend your knees so that your feet are close to your buttocks, but this time spread your legs more than shoulder-width apart. Extend your arms out to the side (fig. 15.1). Inhale.

On the exhale, slowly lower your bent knees to the right until they rest on the ground while simultaneously turning your head fully to the left. This time your left knee should come into contact with the bottom of your right foot. Look at your left hand, then lower both arms so that your left hand touches your left foot and your right hand rests on your right knee (fig. 15.2). Inhale and exhale in place.

On the inhale, return your arms to the T position and slowly raise your knees up while you turn your head back to center (fig. 15.3).

Repeat the asana sequence on the other side.

Key: Gently stretch your legs until both legs come into full contact with the earth.

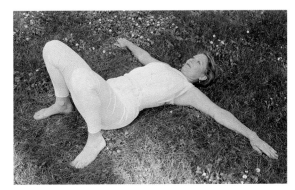

Figure 15.1

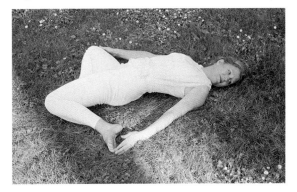

Figure 15.2

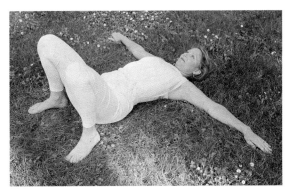

Figure 15.3

Benefits: This asana extends the range of movement in your hips.

Holding the Bridge

Lie on your back, bending your knees until your spine is flat against the ground (fig. 16.1). Keeping your neck and shoulders on the ground, inhale and raise your hips slowly until your back creates a flat

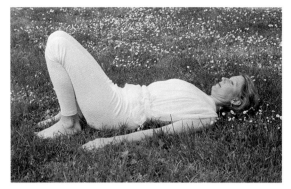

Figure 16.1

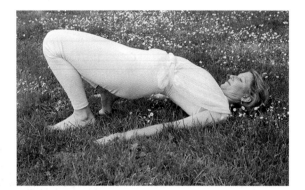

Figure 16.2

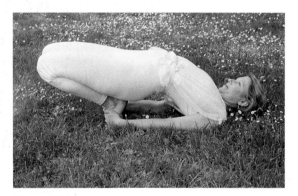

Figure 16.3

while in this position, expanding your belly on the inhalation and leaning slightly forward to stretch your thigh muscles on each exhalation.

To exit the asana, slowly shift weight from left to right legs to ease and lower your spine to the ground. Breathe deeply in a relaxed position for three rounds.

Key: You may want to follow this asana with a forward bend for a counter-stretch—grasping your legs, pull yourself into a fetal position while lying on your back. Breathe deeply.

Benefits: This asana stretches your thigh muscles and your lower back.

The Full Bridge

Lying on your back, bend your elbows and place your hands under your shoulders next to your neck, with your fingers pointing toward your feet. Bend your knees, keeping your feet as close to your buttocks as possible (fig. 17.1). Shift forward slightly, taking most of your body weight on your legs (fig. 17.2). When you feel steady, lift yourself up into a back bend (fig. 17.3). Holding this position, breathe deeply.

When this becomes easy, try slowly turning your head to each side (fig. 17.4).

To end the asana, slowly lower your back to

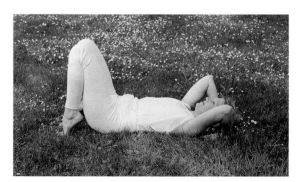

Figure 17.1

plane from your chest to your knees, then move your right foot to underneath your buttock (fig. 16.2). Once your right foot is in place, clasp it with your right hand. Move your left foot back as well, clasping it with your left hand (fig. 16.3). Your head and shoulders should remain on the ground while you place your weight on your bent legs.

Inhale and exhale deeply at least three times

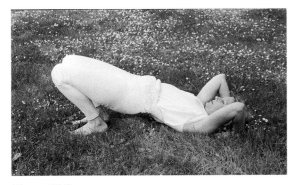

Figure 17.2

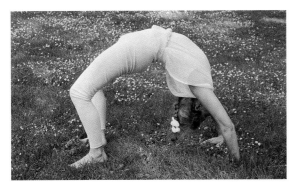

Figure 17.3

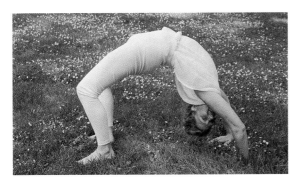

Figure 17.4

the ground. Lie flat on the earth, taking three deep breaths before getting up.

Key: If you are unable to lift yourself up, it is probably because of weakness in the arms or wrists. With practice you may be able to develop these muscles enough to push up.

Benefits: This asana stretches the muscles of the spine and the thigh muscles, and develops upper-body strength.

For the next two asanas, awareness should be centered between the first two chakras, the muladhara and svadisthana, encompassing the region between the anus and the sexual organs and the womb center.

Opening and Closing the Gate

Lie flat on your back with your legs together (fig. 18.1). Inhale. Exhale and raise your straight legs above your head, until you can grasp your calves with your hands (fig. 18.2). On inhale, spread your legs as wide as possible, keeping your legs straight and using your hands to press your legs open (fig. 18.3). On exhale, bend your knees and draw

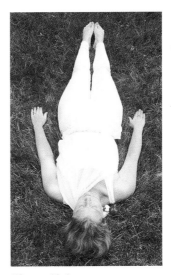

Figure 18.1

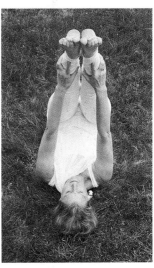

Figure 18.2

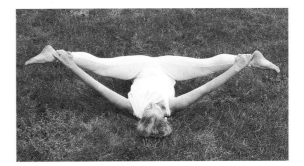

Figure 18.3

THE DANCE OF YOGA * 89

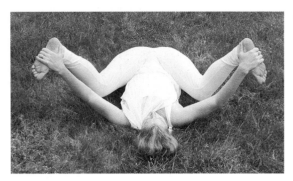

Figure 18.4

them toward you, pulling your legs close to your chest (fig. 18.4). Inhale and straighten your legs to open, then exhale again and pull back.

Repeat this asana four times.

Key: Work your abdominal muscles and draw energy into the womb chakra when you draw your legs toward you.

Benefits: This asana stretches the muscles of the inner thigh.

Triangles

Lying on your back, inhale and extend your legs straight above your head, toes pointed (fig. 19.1). Grasping your right ankle with your right hand and

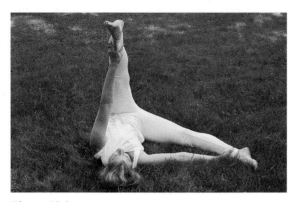

Figure 19.3

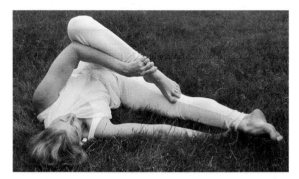

Figure 19.4

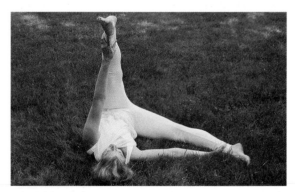

Figure 19.5

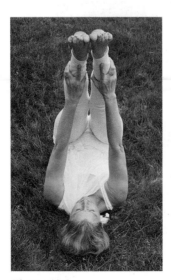

Figure 19.1

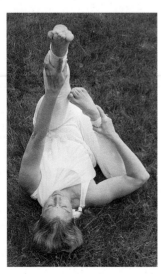

Figure 19.2

left ankle with your left hand, exhale and bend your right knee so that your pointed right toe touches your left knee, and your right knee and thigh are resting on the ground at your right side (fig. 19.2).

Inhale, straightening your right leg so that it is resting fully on the ground (fig. 19.3). Exhaling, bend your left knee and bring your left foot to touch your right knee (fig. 19.4). Inhale and straighten

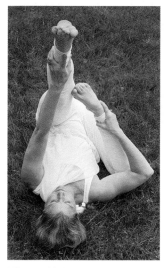
Figure 19.6

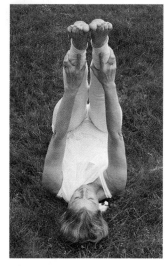
Figure 19.7

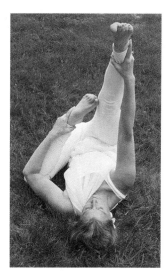
Figure 19.8

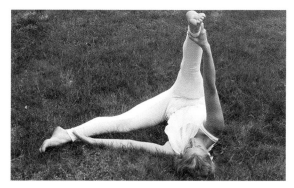
Figure 19.9

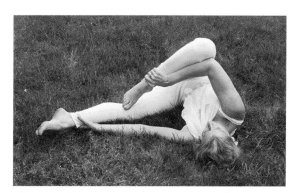
Figure 19.10

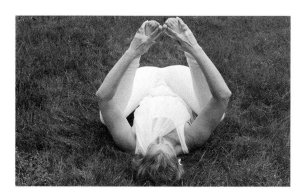
Figure 19.11

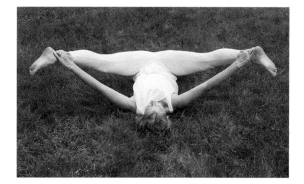
Figure 19.12

both legs once again so that they are at right angles, your right leg on the ground (fig. 19.5).

Bend your right knee once again so that your right foot is touching your left knee (fig. 19.6). Straighten both legs above your head (fig. 19.7).

Repeat the sequence on the left side, this time bending and straightening your left knee (figs. 19.8, 19.9, and 19.10). Now exhale and draw both legs back toward your chest, knees wide apart and toes touching (fig. 19.11). Follow by inhaling and spreading your legs out to the sides (fig. 19.12).

Exhale and straighten your legs up above your head once more. Slowly lower both legs to the ground.

Key: Use your hands grasping your ankles to control the smooth flow of one position into the next.

Benefits: This asana strengthens the lower back and abdomen, and stretches the leg muscles.

The following asana is a simple variation on a spinal twist, performed in a prone position. Beneficial to the shoulders and upper spine, it is especially useful for those who need to proceed gradually into an upper body cross-stretch.

Bent Knee Spinal Twist

Begin by lying on your back with your spine against the earth, knees bent and extended out to the side, the soles of your feet together. Your arms are extended straight out, perpendicular to your body, palms up (fig. 20.1). Inhale and exhale.

Inhale again; on the exhale slowly turn your body to the right, bringing your left arm across your body until it lies on top of your right arm, palms joined, and your left leg rests on top of your

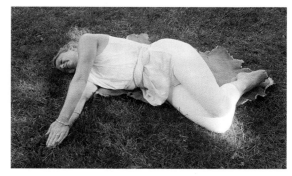

Figure 20.2

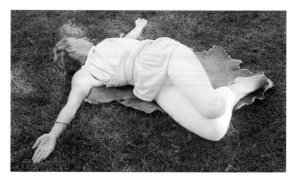

Figure 20.3

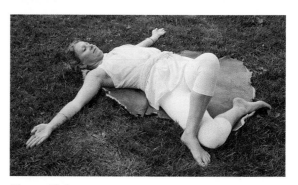

Figure 20.4

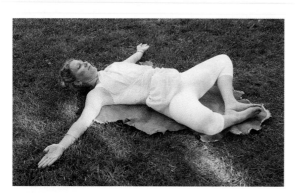

Figure 20.1

right leg (fig. 20.2). Inhale and exhale in place.

On the next inhale, keeping your legs in place and your torso turned to the right, bring your left arm across your body, following it with your eyes. Extend your left arm fully to the left (fig. 20.3). Hold this position and breathe.

On the exhale raise your left leg up and over your right leg, placing your left foot flat on the ground just above your right knee and bringing your focus back to center (fig. 20.4). Hold and

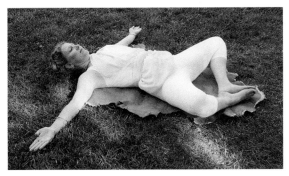

Figure 20.5

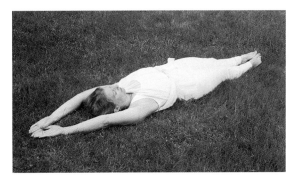

Figure 21.1

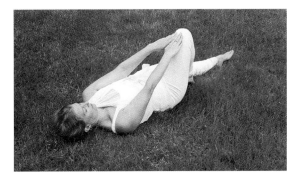

Figure 21.2

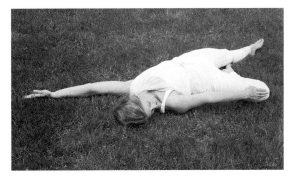

Figure 21.3

breathe. To finish, raise your left leg up and over your right knee and once again join the soles of your feet together, knees out to the side (fig. 20.5).

Repeat the entire sequence on the other side.

Key: When you open your arm out to the side, be sure to keep your opposite knee on the ground. Concentrate on the area between the manipura (the third chakra) and the anahata (the heart center).

Benefits: This asana provides an excellent cross-stretch that benefits the uper back as well as the lower.

This asana, one of my favorites, creates a series of Indian-dance-like still poses when viewed from above. It offers a complete stretch, involving your entire body from head to toe while you remain in full contact with the earth. Concentrating on your third chakra, the pivotal center of your body, perform the asana as a dance, in a slow and fluid cadence, coordinating your movements with your breath.

Horizontal Spinal Twist

Lie flat on your back with your legs together, your arms extended straight up over your head, palms together (fig. 21.1). Inhale.

Exhale, flattening your lower back. Inhale, raising your right knee so that your heel is close to your buttocks. On the exhale, lower both your arms so that your hands rest on your raised right knee (fig. 21.2). Inhale.

Exhale and, keeping your hips on the ground, raise your left hand over your head, placing it at a forty-five-degree angle to the upper left of your torso. With your right hand still on your knee, lower your knee to the floor, keeping your right foot in contact with your left thigh and your right thigh at a right angle to your torso (fig. 21.3). Turn

THE DANCE OF YOGA

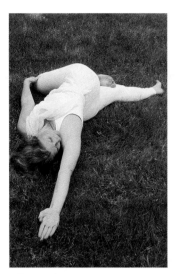

Figure 21.4

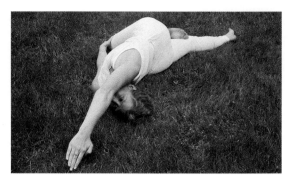

Figure 21.5

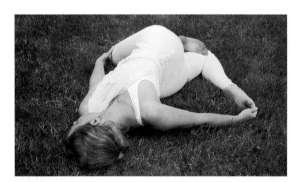

Figure 21.6

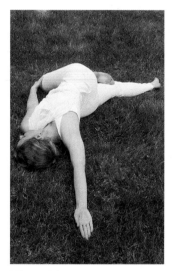

Figure 21.7

your head to the right. Inhale and exhale in place, trying to flatten your spine against the ground.

On the next inhale raise your knee again and, lowering your left arm, hold your right knee with your left hand. Keeping your thigh at a right angle, bring it across your body until your knee touches the ground on your left side (fig. 21.4). Turn your head to the right. Now your right hand is above your head in the forty-five-degree position. Hold this position and slowly inhale and exhale.

On the next exhalation, keeping your hips and lower body in place, turn your upper body and neck in and upward, rotating your right arm diagonally inward until you can look up at your right hand (fig. 21.5). Inhale and exhale in place.

On the next exhale, bend your left knee and bring your fully extended right arm slowly down and around behind you on the ground until you can grasp your left foot with your right hand (fig. 21.6). Inhale and exhale in place.

On the next exhalation, release your left foot and return your hand to the upward position, continuing to face left (fig. 21.7). Inhale. On the exhale slowly face front, raising your right leg and returning it to its original bent-knee position, lowering your arms to place both hands on your knee once more (fig. 21.8). Inhale in place. Exhale and slowly lower your right leg as you lift your arms over your head (fig. 21.9). Inhale and exhale in this position.

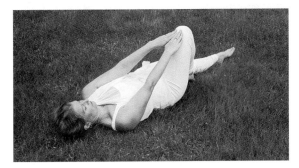

Figure 21.8

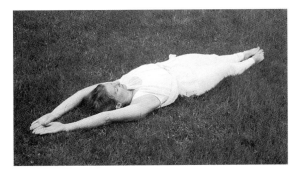

Figure 21.9

Perform the same asana sequence on the other side, lifting your left leg instead of your right and reversing directions.

Key: It may seem a minor detail to turn your head fully to the right or left, but this effectively completes the cross-stretch of the body and produces the best results in this asana.

Benefits: This is an excellent all-over stretch.

Worshiped as the embodiment of the primordial life force, the cobra is India's archetypal sacred serpent. While the cobra moves along the earth on its belly, its flexibility nonetheless renders it capable of lifting itself into an upright position. Hence the snake is associated with Kundalini shakti, the transcendent power that lies dormant at the base of the spine; the ultimate goal of tantric yoga is the enlightenment that occurs when Kundalini rises to the highest level.

The following variation on a classic hatha yoga asana stresses both the dynamic and cyclical nature of the process of all growth and transcendence: Slowly do we begin to escape our limitations and achieve new heights, and often it involves returning again and again to the place from which we began.

The Cobra Cycle

Lie on your belly with your arms stretched out above your head, forehead resting on the earth (fig. 22.1). Slowly inhale, lifting your neck and looking up (fig. 22.2). Exhale and lower your head, bringing your hands back to either side of your face at the level of your ears (fig. 22.3).

Inhale and slowly extend your neck, chin forward, and look up (fig. 22.4). Your abdomen should still be in full contact with the earth, your

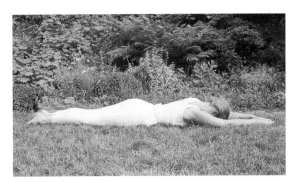

Figure 22.1

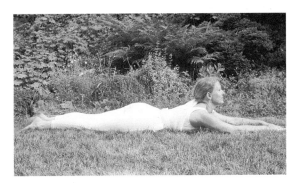

Figure 22.2

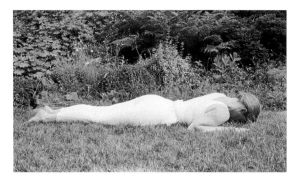

Figure 22.3

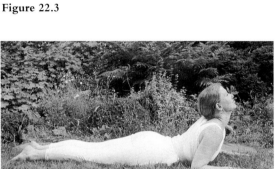

Figure 22.4

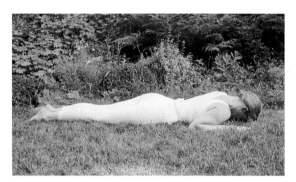

Figure 22.5

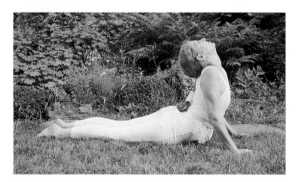

Figure 22.6

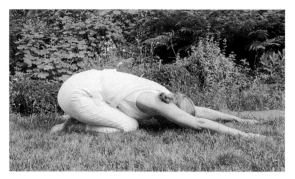

Figure 22.7

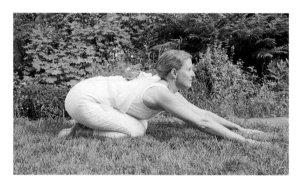

Figure 22.8

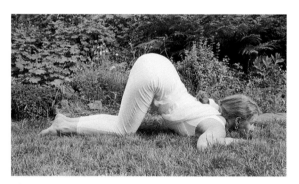

Figure 22.9

shoulders and upper chest lifted. Exhale and slowly lower yourself back down, contracting your abdominal muscles (fig. 22.5).

Inhale and move through the two former positions, lifting yourself until you are finally in full cobra position (fig. 22.6). Be careful to keep your hips on the ground.

On the next exhale, lift your torso up and back until your buttocks are resting on your heels, your

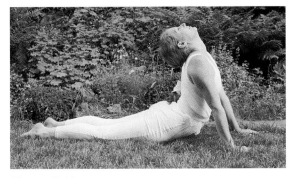

Figure 22.10

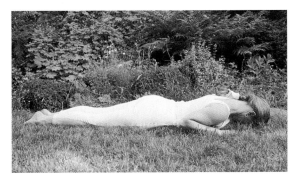

Figure 22.11

head is down, and your arms are extended fully in front of you (fig. 22.7). Inhale and lift your head, expanding your belly (fig. 22.8).

Exhale and, putting weight on your forearms, creep forward with your chest close to the ground until you can rest your knees, chest, and chin on the ground (fig. 22.9). This places the lower spine in a fully concave position. On your next inhale, push forward and up into a full cobra position once more (fig. 22.10). Exhale slowly, gently lowering your body to the ground (fig. 22.11). Extend your arms and rest your full body against the earth to finish.

Key: Perform this asana slowly and deliberately, raising your face chin-first, then raising your neck and shoulders. Similarly on the return, move backward through all the former positions, finally resting your forehead on the ground.

Benefits: This is one of the most effective exercises ever for increasing the flexibility of the spine.

Like the Cobra, the following two asanas involve bending the spine in the same convex direction as the several Bridge asanas described earlier in this section. Notice how different the same stretch feels when, instead of lying on your back, you lie face down.

The Bow

Lie on your belly with your hands stretched over your head, your forehead resting on the earth (fig. 23.1). Inhale. On the exhale, reach back to take hold of your right ankle with your right hand. On the inhale, pull up as if stringing a bow (fig. 23.2). Exhale and slowly release your foot, returning to a prone position (fig. 23.3). Repeat the entire sequence on the left side, pulling up on the left ankle (fig. 23.4).

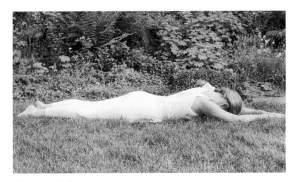

Figure 23.1

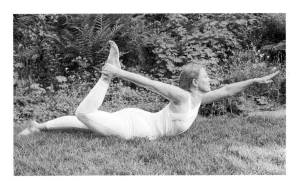

Figure 23.2

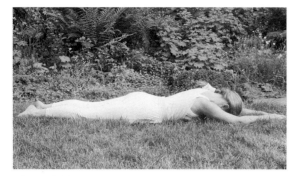

Figure 23.3

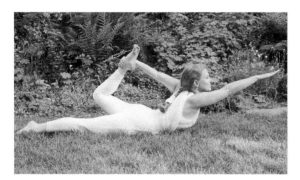

Figure 23.4

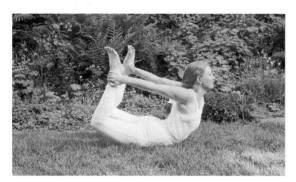

Figure 23.5

After stretching to prone once more, reach back with both hands and pull up into a full bow position (fig. 23.5). Hold and breathe, rocking gently back and forth. Finish with a full stretch and three deep breaths, then relax to prone and breathe.

Key: Hold your ankles from the outside.

Benefits: This asana stretches the muscles of the thighs and increases flexibility of the spine.

To pull yourself up against the force of gravity without using your hands, the following asana requires even more effort than those preceding it. Keep your attention at the womb chakra and breathe as deeply as possible.

Superwoman

Lie on your belly, face down on the earth, with your hands extended out over your head (fig. 24.1). Inhale and exhale in place. On an inhale, raise your legs up behind you and extend your arms out in front (fig. 24.2). Hold this position and breathe in and out without lowering your legs.

To counterbalance this stretch, exhale as you lower your legs to the ground. Inhale in place. On the next exhale, lift your body up and back,

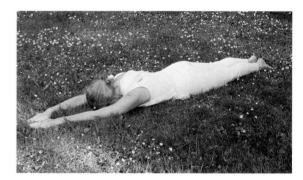

Figure 24.1

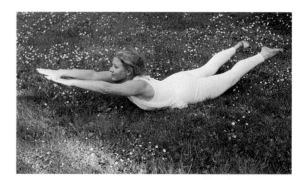

Figure 24.2

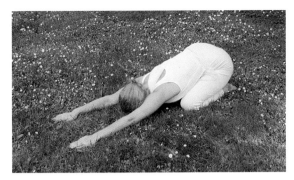

Figure 24.3

until you are finally resting on your haunches (fig 24.3).

Key: Use the muscles of your lower back to do the work.

Benefits: This asana is excellent for toning your abdominal muscles and strengthening your lower back.

Seated Asanas
(Element: Fire)

There is something very basic about sitting on the ground cross-legged. We most often associate yoga with those exercises that are performed while seated on the ground, perhaps because this is the traditional posture for meditation. Seated thus, we remain close to Earth, in touch with her rhythms and energies. At the same time, sitting erect, we express with our bodies the fact that as humans, unlike any other animal, we are not simply "subject to" the earth: We are also transcendent beings. Through the power of our consciousness we rise out of the earth like a plant grows skyward, moving toward a higher awareness of our own nature. In this metaphor the spirit of transcendence is made manifest in the breath. Breathing is the process by which the element of air is transformed into subtle awareness through the element of fire.

Rib Cage Stretch

Sitting on the ground with your back straight and the soles of your feet together, grasp your feet with your hands, keeping your arms straight (fig. 25.1). Inhale and push your lower back slightly inward (fig. 25.2). Now exhale and contract your abdomen, leaning forward with an extended spine until your head is lowered enough to rest on your feet (fig. 25.3). With your head down, inhale and exhale in place.

On your next inhalation contract inward, rolling your spine up into a sitting position (fig. 25.4). Expanding your abdomen, push your spine slightly forward (fig. 25.5). Exhale and contract your abdomen, pushing inward toward your spine as you slide your hands up to your knees and rolling slightly backward until your arms are straight (fig. 25.6).

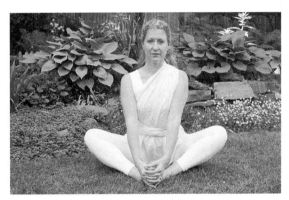

Figure 25.1

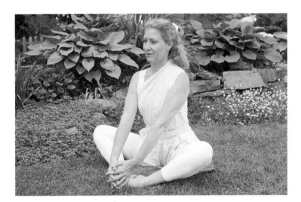

Figure 25.2

THE DANCE OF YOGA ❊ 99

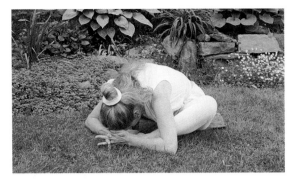

Figure 25.3

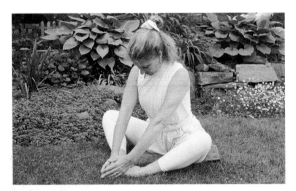

Figure 25.4

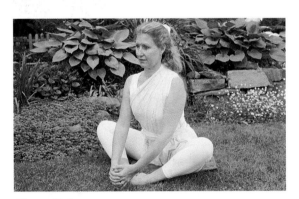

Figure 25.5

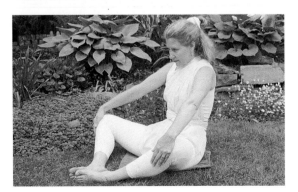

Figure 25.6

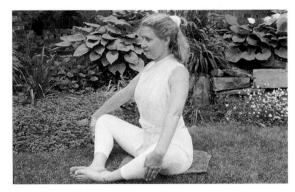

Figure 25.7

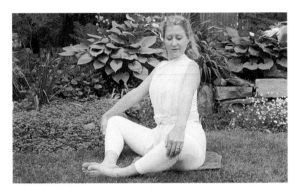

Figure 25.8

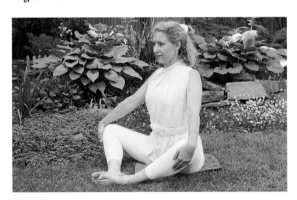

Figure 25.9

Return to a straight sitting position and, inhaling, expand your chest outward, drawing your shoulders back (25.7). Keeping your hands on your knees, on the exhale shift your rib cage to the right and slightly back, turning to look at your left knee (fig. 25.8). Your right arm should be slightly bent while your left arm is straight. Inhale and return to center, chest expanded (25.9).

Exhale and shift your rib cage to the left until

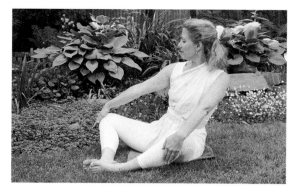

Figure 25.10

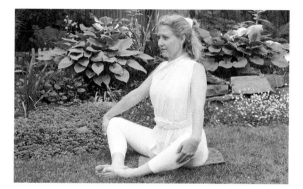

Figure 25.11

the chest. With the incoming and outgoing breaths, feel the energy flow back and forth from the lowest chakras to the heart center.

Graceful Spinal Twists

Begin by sitting with your left heel tucked in close to your pelvis and your right heel resting against your right buttock (fig. 26.1). Your spine should be as straight as possible. Rest your right hand on your right knee and your left hand on your left knee.

On inhale, raise your hands above your head, crossing your wrists and joining your palms (fig. 26.2). On

your right arm is fully extended (fig. 25.10). On the inhale return to center, your chest expanded (fig. 25.11).

Key: In the beginning the range of movement in this exercise may be only a few inches, especially moving right and left. When you reach the limit of your movement, concentrate on expanding and contracting your abdominal muscles, keeping your concentration at the manipura, or womb, chakra.

Benefits: This asana stretches and strengthens the abdominal muscles, affecting the entire waist region, all from a seated position.

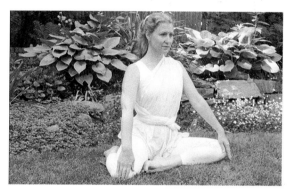

Figure 26.1

For the next three asanas, extend your area of concentration from the womb center downward to the first two chakras at the base of the spine and up to the anahata (heart) chakra, located in the middle of

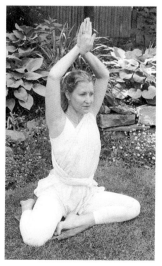

Figure 26.2

THE DANCE OF YOGA ※ 101

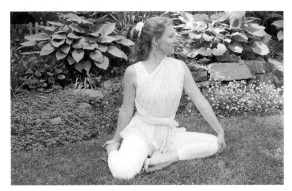

Figure 26.3

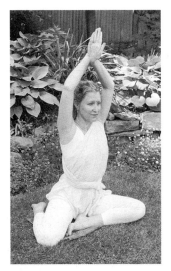

Figure 26.4

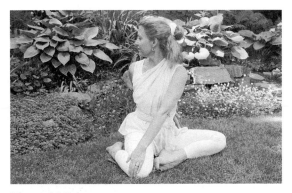

Figure 26.5

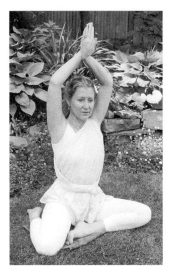

Figure 26.6

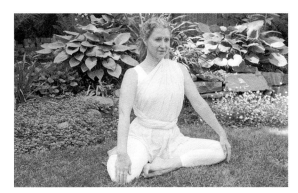

Figure 26.7

exhale, contract your abdomen and extend and lower your arms so that your left hand rests on your left knee and your right hand rests on the bottom of your right foot (fig. 26.3). Turn your face to look over your left shoulder.

On the next inhale, raise your arms over your head again, facing front (fig. 26.4). On exhale, lower your arms so that your left arm rests on your right knee and your right arm wraps around behind your back and grasps your left thigh (or rests on your left hip) (fig. 26.5). On inhale, raise your arms over your head again, facing front (26.6). On exhale, lower your arms to the starting position, right hand on right knee and left hand on left knee (fig. 26.7).

Switch legs and perform the same cycle on the other side, reversing the arm movements.

Key: Keep your lower back straight (tilt your pelvis slightly forward if necessary) and expand and contract your abdominal muscles with all inhalations and exhalations.

Benefits: This exercise trims and firms the waist and increases the flexibility in the lower back, at the same time providing an excellent stretch for your upper arms.

Graceful Spinal Twist Extensions

Begin in a sitting position similar to that in the previous asana, with your left heel tucked into your pelvis; this time extend your right leg out to a forty-five-degree angle in front of you. Inhale and raise your arms above your head, crossing your wrists and joining your palms (fig. 27.1). Exhale and lean up, out, and over your right leg until your head is resting on your right knee (fig. 27.2). Inhale and exhale in place; on the second inhale, rise back up to the sitting position (fig. 27.3).

On the exhale extend your right leg straight out to the side and, still facing front, lean to the right, bending from your waist, to lower your upper body over your leg. At the same time extend your right arm out to hold your leg or your foot and bend your left arm at the elbow to grasp your right elbow with your left hand (fig. 27.4). Inhale

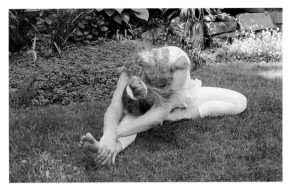

Figure 27.2

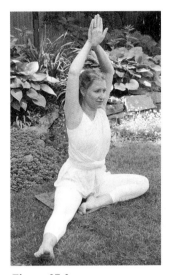

Figure 27.3

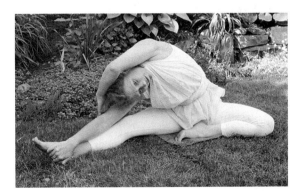

Figure 27.4

and exhale in place, returning to a sitting position on inhale.

Repeat the movement once more, this time extending your right leg forty-five degrees to the

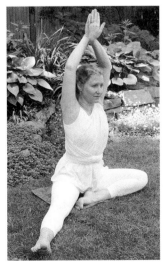

Figure 27.1

THE DANCE OF YOGA ❈ 103

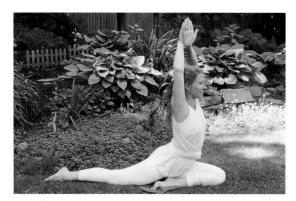

Figure 27.5

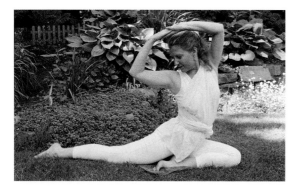

Figure 27.6

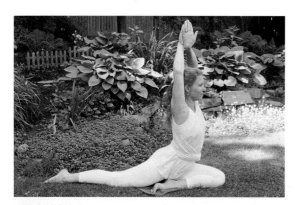

Figure 27.7

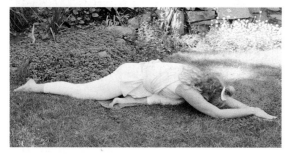

Figure 27.8

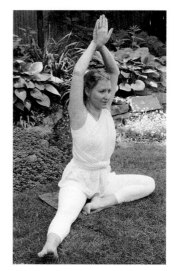

Figure 27.9

back on the exhale and lifting your arms over your head, facing front (fig. 27.5). On the inhale look back over your right leg while rotating your hands, so that your right fingers touch your left palm. Extend your right elbow toward the outstretched leg so that your upper arm is parallel to your leg (fig. 27.6). Hold this position and inhale and exhale.

Raise your arms over your head once more and face front (fig. 27.7). With arms extended, on the exhale lower your upper body down over your left knee (fig. 27.8). Inhale and exhale in place. On an inhale rise up and end by returning your right leg to its starting position (fig. 27.9).

Repeat the entire sequence on the left side.

Key: To create a graceful effect, pull up to elongate your spine as much as possible whenever you raise your hands over your head.

Benefits: This asana stretches your leg muscles and keeps your waist slim and flexible.

Crossover Spinal Twist

Begin this asana with a basic modified lotus posture. Starting from a simple cross-legged sitting posture, bring your left knee forward while you lift

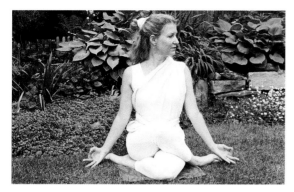

Figure 28.1

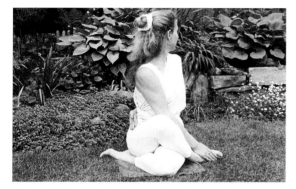

Figure 28.2

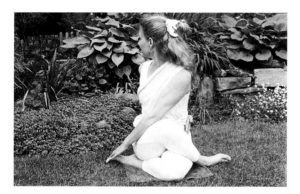

Figure 28.3

On your next exhale slowly turn your body to the left, extending your right hand to meet your right foot and wrapping your left arm around your body until it rests on your right hip (fig. 28.2). Look over your left shoulder. Hold this position and breathe.

On an exhale turn your body slowly in the opposite direction, touching your left foot with your left hand and wrapping your right arm around to rest on your left hip, looking over your right shoulder (fig. 28.3).

To complete the asana, turn to the front and breathe deeply for three rounds. Then perform the entire series with your left leg over your right.

Key: Keep your back as straight as possible while sitting in this position. Be sure to expand on the inhalation and contract when you exhale.

Benefits: This asana stretches the thigh muscles and increases flexibility of the hips.

Seated Cross Stretch

Sit cross-legged with your arms crossed in front of your chest so that your right hand is touching your left knee and your left hand is touching your right knee (fig. 29.1). Keeping your left arm in place, on an inhale raise your right arm above your head in

your right leg and cross it over the left, trying to align your right leg on top of your left as much as possible. Once your right leg is sitting comfortably on top of your left leg, using arala mudra rest your right hand on your left foot and your left hand on your right foot (fig. 28.1). Breathe deeply. Maintaining this posture, turn your head slowly to the right and then the left.

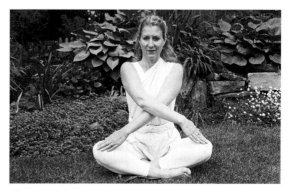

Figure 29.1

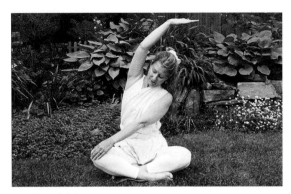

Figure 29.2

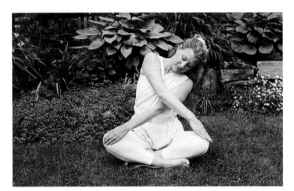

Figure 29.3

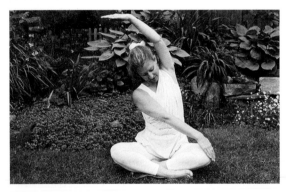

Figure 29.4

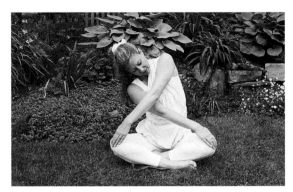

Figure 29.5

Repeat this asana three times on each side.

Key: Pull up at the waist to move the rib cage from side to side.

Benefits: This asana stretches and tones the entire upper body.

The foloowing asana reminds me of the classical depiction of apsaras, *the flying nature spirits of Vedic mythology who dance in the winds and waters. When performing it, use your breath to propel your imagination into magical realms.*

The following three asanas work to strengthen the muscles of the legs, in addition to increasing the flexibility of the spine. When working with the legs, extend your consciousness all the way down to the tips of your toes.

The Extended Rotation

Starting from a cross-legged position, keep your left heel tucked into your pelvis and extend your right leg out to the side. Raise your elbows and place your hands in hamsasya mudra in front of your chest (fig. 30.1) Inhale in place. Exhale and open your arms, changing your hands from hamsasya to alapadma mudra, leaning your upper body to the right until your right hand touches your right foot and your left arm extends behind you on

a graceful line, leaning to the left and looking right (fig. 29.2). On the exhale lower your fully extended right arm to touch your left knee, following the movement with your eyes (fig. 29.3).

Inhale and now raise your left arm, slowly leaning to the right (fig. 29.4). Lower your left arm to your right knee, tracking your moving hand with your eyes (fig. 29.5).

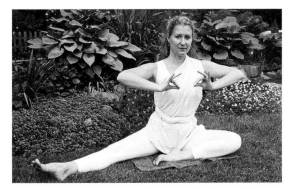

Figure 30.1

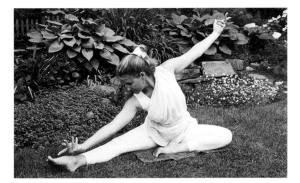

Figure 30.2

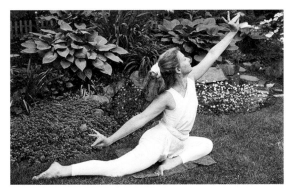

Figure 30.3

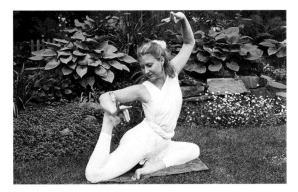

Figure 30.4

the same plane (fig. 30.2). Turn your head to look at your right hand.

Inhale and turn your right knee and hip inward, rotating your arms on the same plane, moving your hands back into hamsasya mudra while looking up at your left hand (fig. 30.3). Inhale in place. On the exhale, turning back to look at your right foot, bend your right knee and wrap your right arm around your right ankle, bending your left arm up over your head (fig. 30.4). Hold this position and breathe.

Work your way back to the beginning by going through each of the positions in the reverse order. Repeat the sequence on the left side.

Key: Stretch your arms out fully in the open position, rotating your forearm when changing from hamsasya to alapadma mudra but keeping your shoulders as relaxed as possible.

Benefits: This asana stretches the upper back, neck, and shoulders, as well as the hips and legs.

Back Leg Rotation Cycle

Begin by sitting with your left leg tucked behind you so that your left heel touches your buttocks while you extend your right leg out to the side. Grasp your right toe with your right hand and rest your left hand on your left foot behind you (fig. 31.1). On the exhale, stretch forward until you can rest your head on your right knee (fig. 31.2).

Inhale to sit up and lean back, placing your left hand behind your left buttock. Raise yourself up to balance on your left knee and right heel, extending your right arm up and back over your head so that it is in a straight line with your right leg (fig. 31.3). Exhale to come down into your original seated position (fig. 31.4). Finish by bringing your joined palms together in front of your chest.

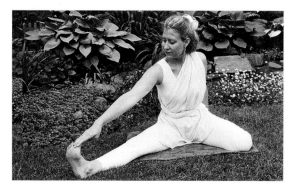

Figure 31.1

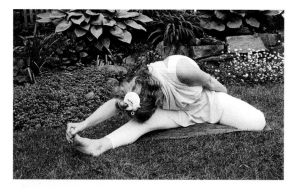

Figure 31.2

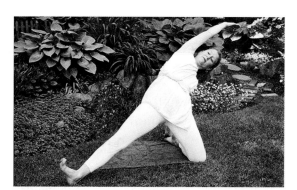

Figure 31.3

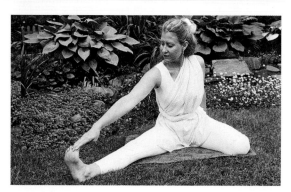

Figure 31.4

Repeat this sequence three times on each side.

Key: Try to keep your extended leg as straight as possible when you stretch down to rest your head on your knee.

Benefits: This asana stretches the lower back and the tendons in the back of the legs.

The Full Extension

To reach the first position of this next asana cycle, sit with your right leg tucked into your pelvis and your left leg extended out to the side (fig. 32.1). Placing your hands on either side of you, turn and shift your weight so that you are sitting on your right leg, your heel resting alongside the inside of your left thigh (fig. 32.2). Once you are in position, push your chest forward and straighten your

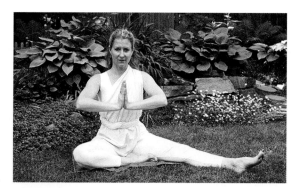

Figure 32.1

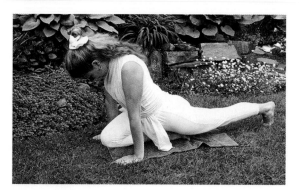

Figure 32.2

back, looking to the front and joining your palms in front of your chest (fig. 32.3). Make sure to keep your elbows raised. Inhale and exhale in place.

Inhale again. On the exhale turn your body to the left, straightening your arms and opening your hands into alapadma mudra (fig. 32.4). Your left arm will extend down and back toward your left foot, while your right arm will extend upward on a diagonal along the same plane. Look back at your left hand. Inhale in place. Exhale and return to the frontal position (fig. 32.5).

Now exhale and extend your arms in the opposite direction, your left arm extended upward and in front of you at a forty-five-degree angle, your right arm extended backward toward the left leg on the same plane, with your hands now in hamsasya mudra (fig. 32.6). Look back at your right hand. Inhale in place. On exhale, return to the frontal position (fig. 32.7).

Inhale and raise your hands above your head, palms still joined (fig. 32.8). Exhale and lower your joined palms to the ground, keeping your arms straight and lowering your head until your forehead rests on the ground (fig. 32.9). Inhale and exhale in place. Inhale and raise your spine to sitting position, your palms joined in front of your chest (fig. 32.10).

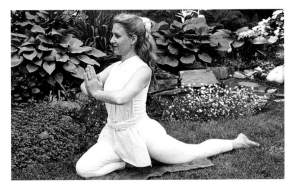

Figure 32.3

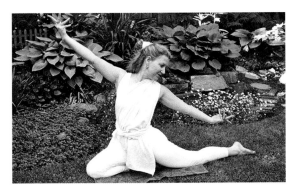

Figure 32.4

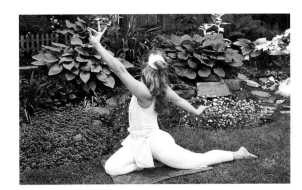

Figure 32.6

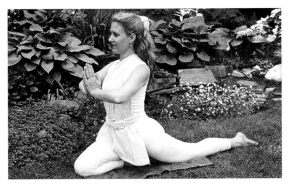

Figure 32.5

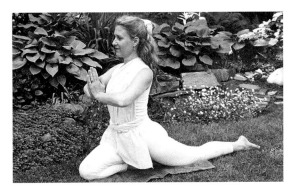

Figure 32.7

THE DANCE OF YOGA

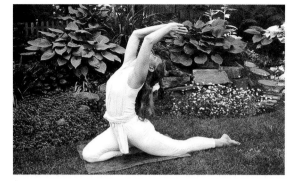

Figure 32.8

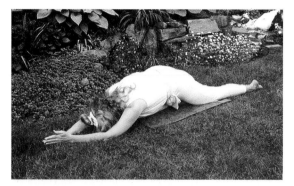

Figure 32.9

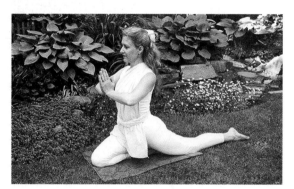

Figure 32.10

Repeat the entire asana sequence on the opposite side.

Key: Focus on the pivotal point of balance, which in this posture is quite low in the body—around the womb center or third chakra area. Try to concentrate on this area while performing the movements.

Benefits: This asana develops strength in the legs and overall balance.

I call this asana the Odd Fish because it is my own variation on the classic fish yoga asana, which is usually performed with the legs fully extended. Concentration should be kept at the third chakra, just below the navel.

The Odd Fish

Begin by sitting on your knees with your legs slightly apart, your hands resting on your thighs in arala mudra, palms up (fig. 33.1). Your spine should be as straight as possible. Inhale and exhale in this position. Inhale again; on the exhale place

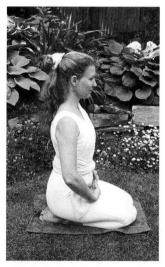

Figure 33.1

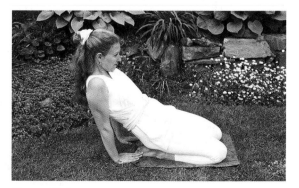

Figure 33.2

your hands on either side of you behind your feet, palms facing forward. Slowly shift your weight backward onto your hands, lowering your chin onto your chest (fig. 33.2). Inhale and arch your back, lifting your pelvis upward and bending your neck completely backward, your hands turned toward the front (fig. 33.3).

Exhale and slowly lower your forearms to the ground, shifting your weight gently backward onto your arms and lowering your head backward so that your neck is fully extended and the top of your head is resting on the ground (fig. 33.4). Inhale deeply and expand your lungs; exhale and contract your abdominal muscles.

Taking the full weight on your forearms, lift your neck gently, then shift farther back until your weight is resting on your shoulders and your back is on the ground (fig. 33.5). Inhale and exhale, lowering your arms to either side of your body, hands in arala mudra once more. On the exhale try to flatten your lower back against the ground. Hold this position and breathe for as long as you comfortably can.

To return to the starting position, on an exhale raise your body back onto your forearms and move backward through each of the former positions

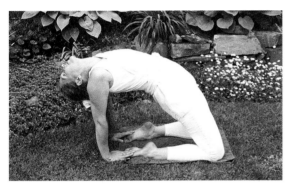

Figure 33.3

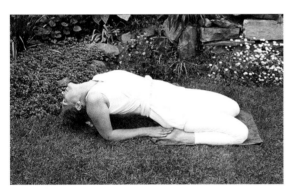

Figure 33.4

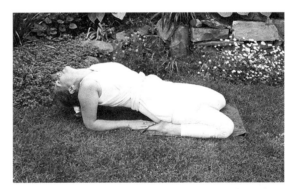

Figure 33.6

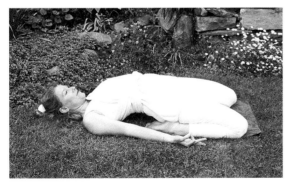

Figure 33.5

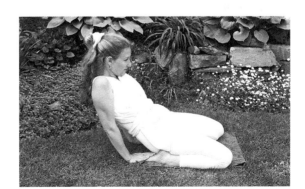

Figure 33.7

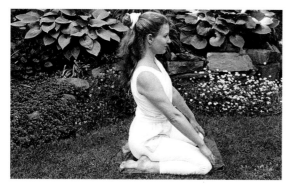

Figure 33.8

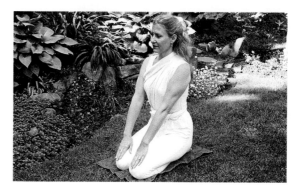

Figure 34.1

(figs. 33.6, 33.7, and 33.8). Be careful to change your position during the exhalations.

Key: Be sure to move slowly when you are raising and lowering your head, to avoid straining your neck.

Benefits: This asana stretches the lower back, as well as the thighs and calves.

Spinal Stretch Cycle

Sit on your knees with your legs together, arms relaxed, your hands resting palm down on each thigh (fig. 34.1). On the inhale, lift your arms and raise your body up until you are "standing" on your knees, your hands extended over your head, palms together (fig. 34.2). Exhale and lean forward with your arms outstretched until your hands touch the ground, your body extended as far forward as possible (fig. 34.3). Your face will be close to the ground, your buttocks raised up, and your lower back will be nearly straight.

Inhale, lowering your forearms to rest on the ground while lifting your head and looking up (fig. 34.4). Here your body will shift slightly forward. Expand your abdominal muscles on inhale and work your upper back muscles by flexing your spine into a concave position. Exhale, straightening your back and dropping your head, contracting your abdominal muscles and shifting your body backward

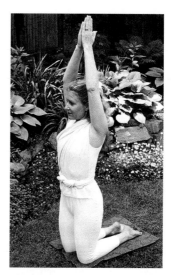

Figure 34.2

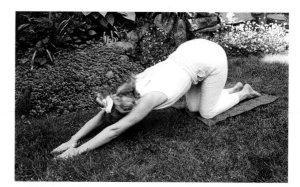

Figure 34.3

so that your buttocks rest on your heels (fig. 34.5).

Inhale and lift your head, returning your back to a concave position, forearms on the ground (fig. 34.6). Exhale and lower your head, lifting

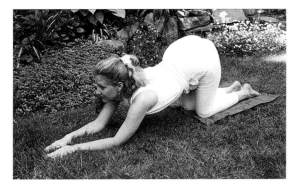

Figure 34.4

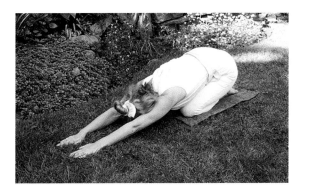

Figure 34.5

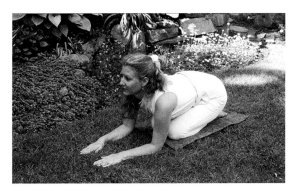

Figure 34.6

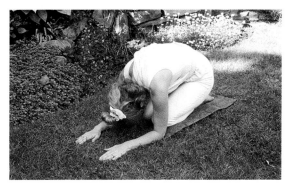

Figure 34.7

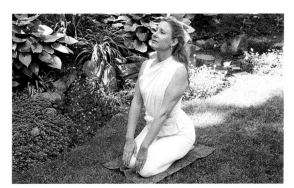

Figure 34.8

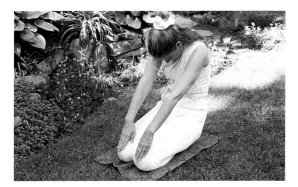

Figure 34.9

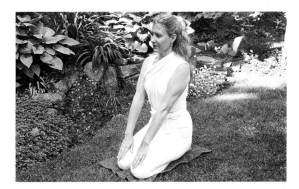

Figure 34.10

your buttocks a few inches in order to fully contract your abdominal muscles (fig. 34.7). Inhale and raise up, hands on your knees, pushing your lower back forward (fig. 34.8). Exhale, shifting your weight back and curving your back to make a convex shape, lowering your head between straightened arms, palms resting on your knees (fig. 34.9). Inhale, slowly raising your head to the beginning sitting position (fig. 34.10).

Key: Be sure to perform this asana as slowly as possible, concentrating on your breathing.

Benefits: This asana provides an even more thorough stretch than the Cobra, as it stretches and contracts the muscles and nerves at several points along the spine.

This is my variation of the Camel, a hatha yoga classic. The camel has tremendous stamina because it knows how to conserve energy: by moving slowly and methodically it can survive incredibly long journeys into the desert. Similarly, by practicing this asana slowly and regularly you will steadily increase your lung capacity and stamina.

The Shifting Camel

Begin kneeling, legs slightly apart (fig 35.1). On an inhale, raise your body so that you are standing on your knees, arms stretched overhead, palms together (fig. 35.2). Exhale in place. Inhale; on exhale, bend backward and to the right, your right hand taking hold of your right ankle (fig. 35.3).

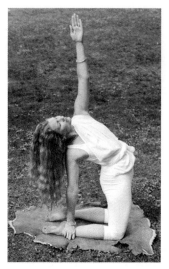

Figure 35.3

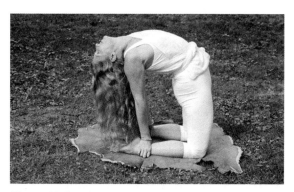

Figure 35.4

Your left arm remains extended overhead. Hold this position and breathe.

On an exhale bend backward, extending your head behind you and lowering your left arm to take hold of your left ankle (fig. 35.4). Hold this position and breathe for three rounds. Now release your right hand and extend your right arm over your head, shifting your weight to your left arm and looking up at your right hand (fig. 35.5).

To return to the knee-standing position let go of your left ankle and, using the muscles of your back, pull yourself up so that your spine is straight once more, your palms joined above your head (fig. 35.6). Repeat the entire sequence beginning on the left side.

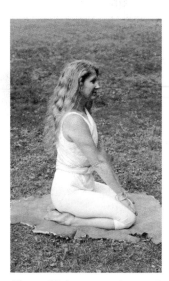

Figure 35.1

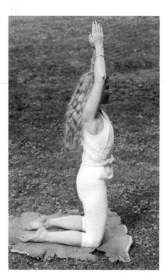

Figure 35.2

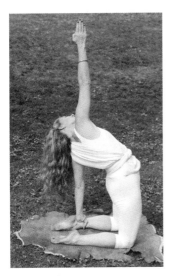

Figure 35.5

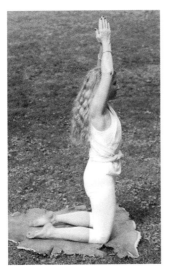

Figure 35.6

Key: Be sure to move on the exhale as directed. Retain control over all your muscles, especially the neck.

Benefits: This asana is excellent for drawing energy into the third chakra and the entire solar plexus area, and for increasing the flexibility of the spine.

❋

The following asana invokes the spirit of the nagini, the female serpent goddess, one of the most ancient archetypes of Indian religion. Snakes are universally worshiped as sacred in Hinduism, and even today in tribal areas women become possessed by the spirits of snakes and dance with loosened hair and wild abandon. This is a tame version of the basic movement they use to express this powerful earth energy.

The Nagini

Begin by sitting on your knees, your spine straight, hands raised above your head with palms side by side, fingers slightly bent to form sarpasirsa mudra (fig. 36.1). On the inhale lift up off your knees, pushing your lower spine forward into a concave position. With your arms and hands still raised and your shoulders back, pull your elbows back as far as possible and tilt your hands forward (fig. 36.2). Continue the inhale as you tilt your head back, moving your pelvis forward and placing your entire spine in a fully concave position, straightening your wrists to point your hands up and back (fig. 36.3). This inhale is long, and the movement continuous.

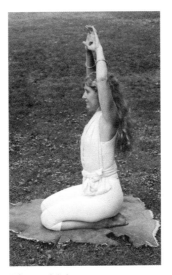

Figure 36.1

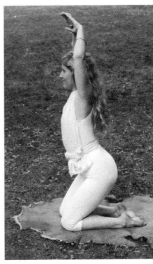

Figure 36.2

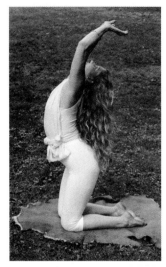
Figure 36.3

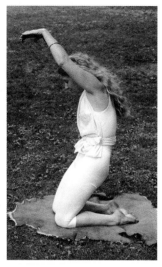
Figure 36.4

Benefits: The Nagini gives the spine an excellent, fluid stretch.

I can never perform the following asana without remembering the story told to me by an Indian woman friend. When she was a little girl her sister and she found a book of asanas in her parent's library. It soon became a favorite activity of theirs to terrify each other with the photo of Sinhasana, the Lion pose. Scary as it can look, this pose has many benefits for the vishuddha chakra, in the region of the throat.

The Lioness

Sitting on your knees, inhale and exhale deeply (fig. 37.1). Inhale once more, filling your lungs completely. Lean forward and, with your fingers extended, place your weight on your arms. Exhale forcefully, opening your eyes and mouth as wide as possible; make an "AAAH" sound as you thrust your tongue out (fig. 37.2). To finish, sit back on your knees and relax, breathing deeply (fig. 37.3).

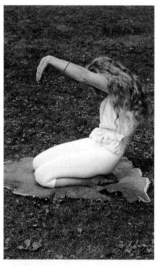
Figure 36.5

On the exhale move in a flowing way downward, back into the seated posture, gradually bringing your spine into a convex position and your hands forward (fig. 36.4). Still exhaling, as you reach the seated posture move your spine into a fully convex position by leaning forward and looking down, hands still slightly overhead, elbows back (fig. 36.5).

Repeat this asana three times without stopping.

Key: This asana should be performed as a continuously flowing movement.

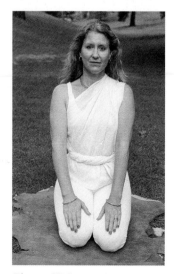
Figure 37.1

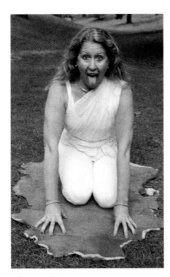

Figure 37.2

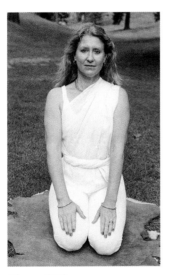

Figure 37.3

Key: Don't be inhibited. Everyone looks strange while performing this one.

Benefits: This asana draws energy into the eyes, ears, and throat. It increases circulation to the facial muscles, and is a good exercise for releasing pent-up emotion.

※

The following asana is named for the female sexual organ, which in Hinduism is revered as the source of creation. Of all the seated asanas, this one encourages the greatest opening of the entire pelvic area. When performing it, concentration should be kept at the lowest two chakras, between the anus and sexual organs.

The Yoni

Sit with the soles of your feet and the palms of your hands joined, your back straight (fig. 38.1). Inhale in place. Exhale and, stretching from the lower spine, lean all the way forward, weaving your arms under your legs and grasping your feet with your hands, palms in (fig. 38.2). Lean forward until your head is resting on your feet. Inhale and exhale in place.

On your next inhale, raise your upper body slightly, lifting your head and still grasping your

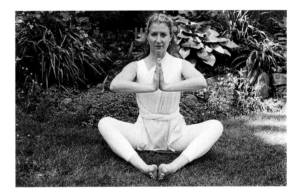

Figure 38.1

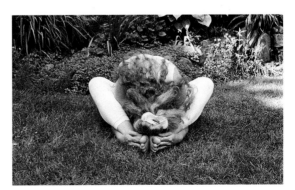

Figure 38.2

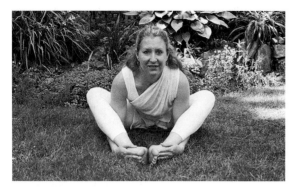

Figure 38.3

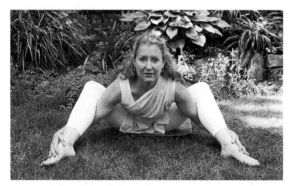

Figure 38.4

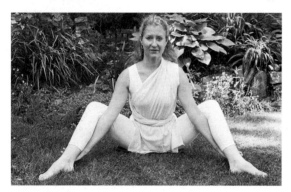

Figure 38.5

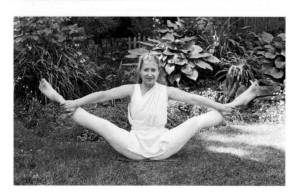

Figure 38.6

feet (fig. 38.3). Exhale in place. Inhale and spread your legs to the side, knees bent, your feet on the ground and your hands still wrapped around your legs (fig. 38.4). Exhale in place.

On the inhale sit up even farther and open your legs out even more, lifting your knees higher (fig. 38.5). Sit as straight as possible, trying to straighten your spine. Exhale in place. Finally, holding your ankles, straighten your legs up and out to the side (fig. 38.6). Hold and breathe in this position for as long as you can.

To complete this asana lower your legs slowly to the ground, return to the starting position, and breathe deeply three times.

Key: Use control over your lower back muscles to balance in the final open-leg position.

Benefits: This asana stretches your entire back from the lower spine, and stretches your legs while developing balance.

Being the slightly wild creatures they are, most yoginis love to rock and roll (especially when it offers a massage to the spine). When practicing this asana, be sure to use a soft yoga mat or rug to cushion the bones of your spine against the hard ground. If you are practicing outside, soft grass works best.

The Spinal Rock and Roll

Begin by sitting with your back straight, your knees bent, your hands resting on your knees (fig. 39.1). Roll backward all the way up to your shoulders and neck (figs. 39.2 and 39.3). Using your legs to "pump" and propel yourself, rock forward, back into the seated posture (fig. 39.4). Inhale as you rock back and exhale as you rock forward.

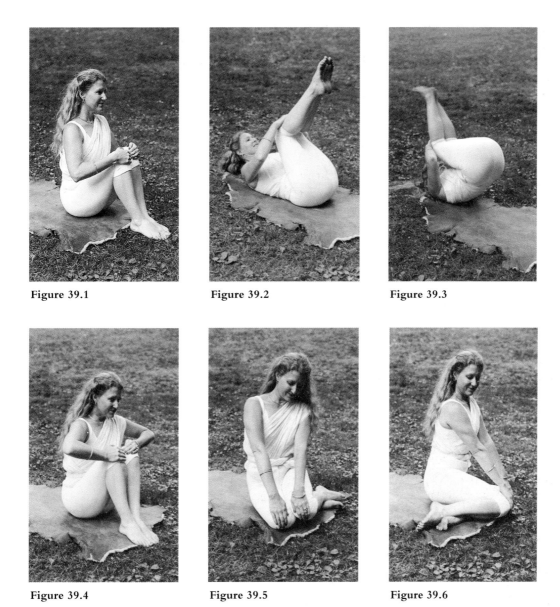

Figure 39.1 **Figure 39.2** **Figure 39.3**

Figure 39.4 **Figure 39.5** **Figure 39.6**

Repeat, this time rolling slightly to the side on the forward roll and pushing both knees on the ground when you reach the seated position (fig. 39.5). Hold for a few seconds and then rock back again, this time twisting to the other side on the forward roll (fig. 39.6).

Repeat each movement at least four times, then return to the seated position.

Key: Contract your spine to expose the muscle and bone when you rock backward and roll sideways.

Benefits: This is a great asana for awakening the spine in the morning.

Arm Movements
(Element: Water)

The arms provide the lyricism of Indian classical dance. The mudras, or hand positions, are carried by the arms; therefore the gracefulness of the arms and upper-body carriage provide the central focus of the "language" of the dance. As the arms are mostly held perpendicular to the torso, the discipline of Indian dance naturally tones the arms and upper body.

The following asanas are based on the arm movements of Indian dance and lead to the same beneficial results. They are also a lot of fun to perform as you concentrate on the position of the hands, wrists, and elbows, all the way down to the fingertips.

As these asanas are performed while seated in a cross-legged position, the center of your awareness may be placed at the anahata chakra, or heart center. Like water, let the movements of your arms flow gently from the heart, the center of your emotions.

Pressing the Palms

On inhale raise your hands over your head, palms together, elbows apart (fig. 40.1). Press your palms together with force. Exhale and lower your right elbow straight down, still pressing palms together (fig. 40.2). Inhale and raise the same elbow up again, releasing tension.

Exhale and lower your left elbow (fig. 40.3). Inhale and raise.

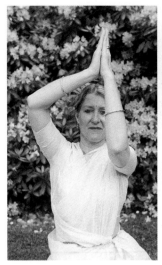
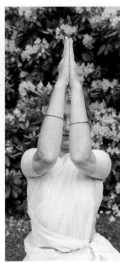

Figure 40.3 **Figure 40.4**

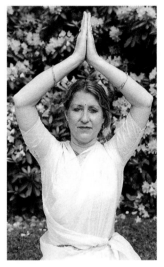

Figure 40.5

Exhale and lower both your elbows until they meet (fig. 40.4). Inhale and lift both your elbows (fig. 40.5). Exhale and lower your joined palms to the level of your forehead (fig. 40.6). Inhale and press your palms together. Exhale and lower your right elbow (fig. 40.7). Inhale and raise it, then exhale and lower your left elbow (fig. 40.8).

Inhale and raise both elbows. Lower both elbows on the exhale (fig. 40.9).

Inhale and raise both elbows overhead. On exhale, lower your joined palms in front of

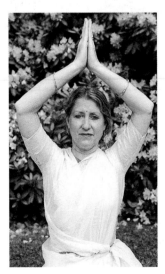
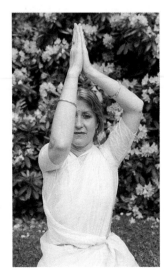

Figure 40.1 **Figure 40.2**

120 ☙ THE DANCE OF YOGA

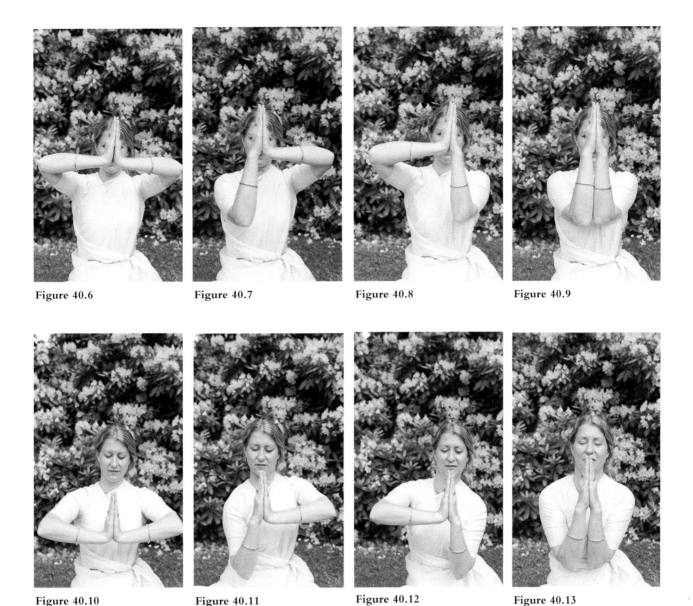

Figure 40.6 Figure 40.7 Figure 40.8 Figure 40.9

Figure 40.10 Figure 40.11 Figure 40.12 Figure 40.13

your chest (fig. 40.10). Repeat the former movements, lowering first one elbow, then the other, and then both (figs. 40.11, 40.12, and 40.13). Each time, bring your arms back to the raised-elbow position.

Key: Maintain as much pressure as possible while pressing your palms together.

Benefits: This exercise provides the same benefits as weight lifting—better muscle tone in the arms and chest—without the use of weights.

Parallel Pulls

Inhale and raise your hands over your head, holding your left forefinger with your right hand (fig. 41.1). Without moving your neck, look upward toward your hands.

On exhale, bend your right elbow and lower your right arm until your upper arm extends straight out from your shoulder; turn your head completely to the right (fig. 41.2).

Inhale and raise your hands over your head

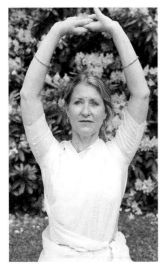
Figure 41.1

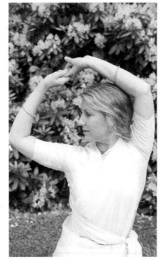
Figure 41.2

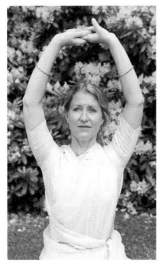
Figure 41.3

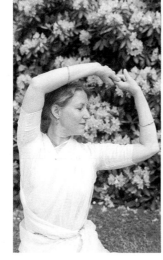
Figure 41.4

ground, your hands in hamsasya mudra (fig. 42.1). Keeping your left hand where it is, inhale and raise your right hand above your head, opening your hand into alapadma mudra (fig. 42.2). Exhale and return to the starting position (fig. 42.3). For the duration of the asana, each time you extend your arm open your hand into alapadma mudra, and each time you return to the starting position move your hand back into hamsasya mudra.

Inhale and move your arm to the upper-right forty-five-degree position (fig. 42.4). Exhale and return your arm to its starting position. Now inhale and extend your arm fully to the right,

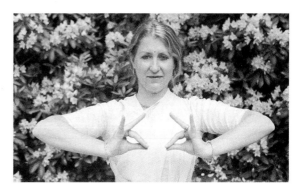
Figure 42.1

again (fig. 41.3). Exhale and extend your arms to the left side (fig. 41.4).

Key: For maximum benefit, pull your arms in opposite directions to keep pressure on your muscles.

Benefits: This asana stretches and tones the forearms and upper arms.

Arm Extensions

Seated on the ground, begin by placing your hands in front of your chest, your arms parallel to the

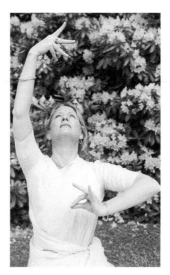
Figure 42.2

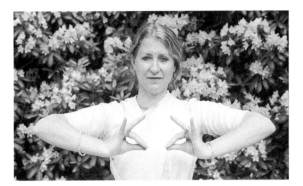

Figure 42.3

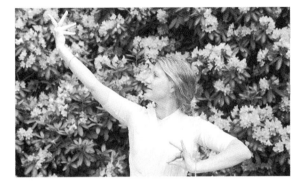

Figure 42.4

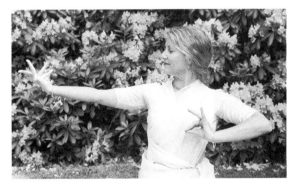

Figure 42.5

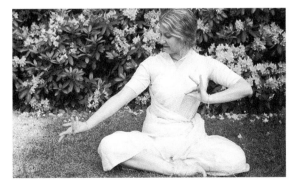

Figure 42.6

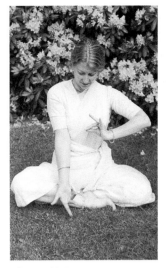

Figure 42.7

forming a straight line with your arm and looking to the right (fig. 42.5). Exhale and return to the starting position.

On the next inhalation bring your arm to the lower-right forty-five-degree position (fig. 42.6). Once again, exhale to return to the starting position. Finally, inhale to a fully extended lower position (fig. 42.7). Exhale back to the starting position.

Repeat the entire sequence using your left arm.

Key: Keep your elbows raised at all times. As you watch your hand, move your head only as much as necessary to keep the hand that is being extended in sight. Consciously contract the muscles of your arm while extending your hand.

Benefits: This asana stretches and tones your arms all the way down to your fingertips.

Double Arm Extensions

Sit cross-legged with your hands in hamsasya mudra in front of your chest, your elbows raised so that your arms are parallel to the ground (fig. 43.1). Inhale and raise both your arms straight above your head, opening your fingers into alapadma mudra (fig. 43.2). Exhale and, keeping your arms fully

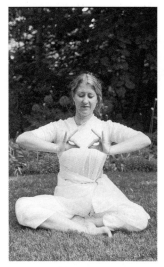

Figure 43.1

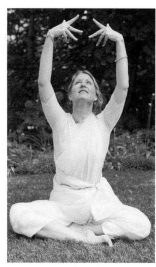

Figure 43.2

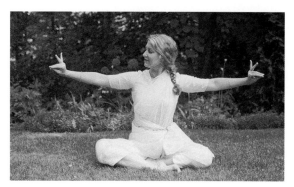

Figure 43.5

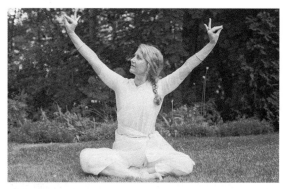

Figure 43.3

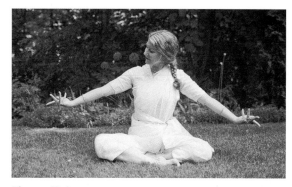

Figure 43.6

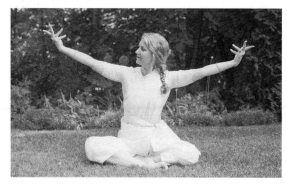

Figure 43.4

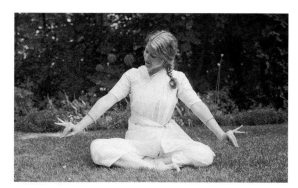

Figure 43.7

extended, turn your wrists and arms over and move your fingers back into hamsasya mudra (fig. 43.3). Inhale and turn your arms, still fully extended, into alapadma mudra (fig. 43.4).

Alternate between hamsasya mudra and ala-

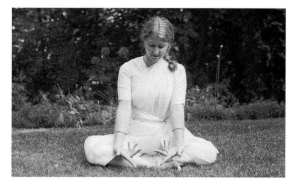

Figure 43.8

124 » THE DANCE OF YOGA

padma mudra, moving fully extended arms downward in a circle until both your arms are fully extended toward the floor (figs. 43.5–43.8). Exhale and return to the starting position.

Key: Keep the muscles of your arms as taut as possible by working with completely straight arms. Be sure to keep your elbows lifted.

Benefits: This asana develops the muscles in both the front and back of the arms.

The Figure Eight

In seated posture, raise your right elbow so that your upper arm is parallel to the ground, your hand in alapadma mudra (fig. 44.1). Inhaling, turn your forearm up and back so that your palm faces upward. Leading with the outer edge of your

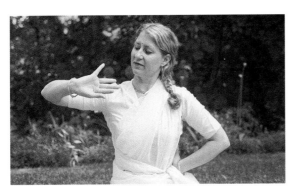

Figure 44.1

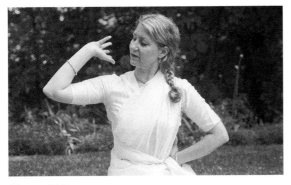

Figure 44.2

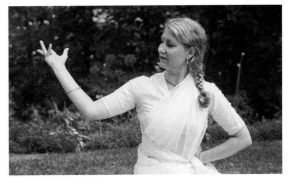

Figure 44.3

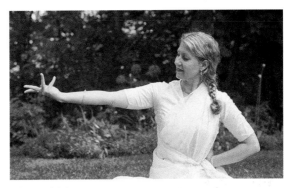

Figure 44.4

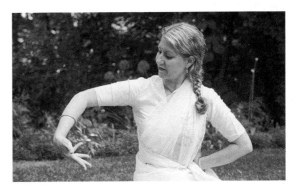

Figure 44.5

palm, move your hand back and out over your shoulder, until your arm is fully extended (figs. 44.2, 44.3, and 44.4).

As soon as your arm reaches the extended position, exhale and turn the palm downward. Still leading with the outer edge of the palm, move your hand down and under your upper arm, and extend it backward as far as you can without dropping the elbow (figs. 44.5, 44.6, and 44.7). Be sure to keep your elbow raised. Once you have

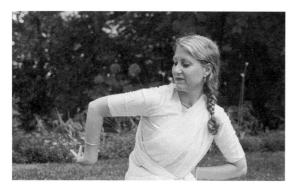

Figure 44.6

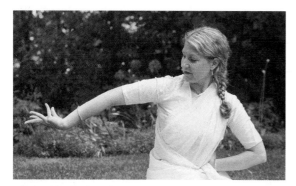

Figure 44.7

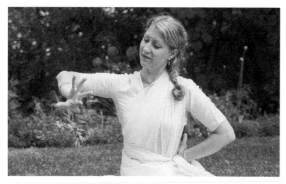

Figure 44.8

uous movement in which you regulate your breath according to the speed of the movement. Begin with large movements with your arm fully extended, and then narrow the movement by working the wrist more and keeping the elbow stationary.

Benefits: One of the favorite asanas of my women's yoga class, this is a demanding but excellent exercise for strengthening the arms, as it alternately extends and then contracts the muscles in a rotating motion.

The Wave

Seated in a cross-legged position, gracefully raise your right arm from the elbow and shift your rib cage by leaning slightly to the right. Turn your head to the right so that you are looking at your right hand (fig. 45.1). To the extent that you raise your right elbow your left elbow correspondingly sinks, but your left hand remains facing upward.

In a slow, continuous movement like a wave, let your elbows rise and fall. As one elbow sinks, the other elbow rises (figs. 45.2, 45.3, and 45.4). The forearm is kept very soft, not rigid, and the hand on each side follows the elbow. Watch each hand as it rises and falls, shifting your weight, and your gaze, from right to left.

extended your arm as fully as possible, continue moving it outward and upward until you reach the starting position and begin to inhale (fig. 44.8).

If kept moving continuously, your arm will create a kind of over-and-under motion that can be performed at various speeds. Practice first with your right arm and then with your left.

Key: This asana should be performed as a contin-

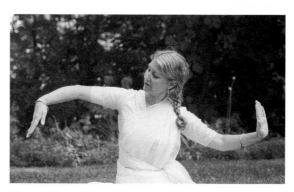

Figure 45.1

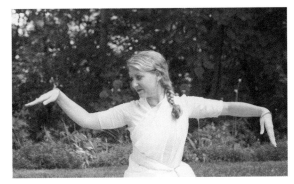

Figure 45.2

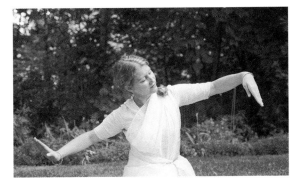

Figure 45.3

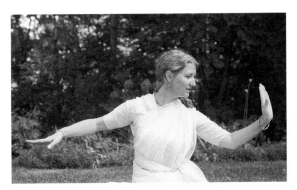

Figure 45.4

Key: As with the previous asana, perform this one as a continuous motion and regulate your breath to the slow tempo of the movement. Remain mobile at the waist as you shift your weight from side to side. Keep your arms and shoulders fully relaxed, performing the movement primarily from the elbows.

Benefits: This asana is a good counterbalance to the Figure Eight. It relaxes the arms and increases flexibility in the shoulders.

Eye and Neck Movements
(Elements: Air and Space)

Nothing is more distinctive about Indian dance than its extensive use of eye movements, which are employed in both pure dance (nritta) to bring attention to the movement in other parts of the body, and in lyrical dance (nritya) to convey emotional content. Neuro-linguistic programming techniques demonstrate that the movement of the eyes indicates that we are accessing various areas of the brain in the search for stored information. By practicing a full range of eye movement we therefore stimulate various nerve endings inside the brain, which encourages mental alertness and holistic patterns of thought.

Awareness therefore centers on the upper chakras, between the fifth and sixth—the area between vishuddha, the throat center, and ajna, the "third eye" in the middle of the forehead. Energy is then automatically transmitted to the sahasrara, or topmost chakra, corresponding to the brain.

Eye Exercises

In a seated position, spine relaxed but upright, bring your attention to your eyes. Look up, feeling the muscles of the eyes as you do so (fig. 46.1).

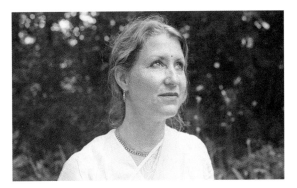

Figure 46.1

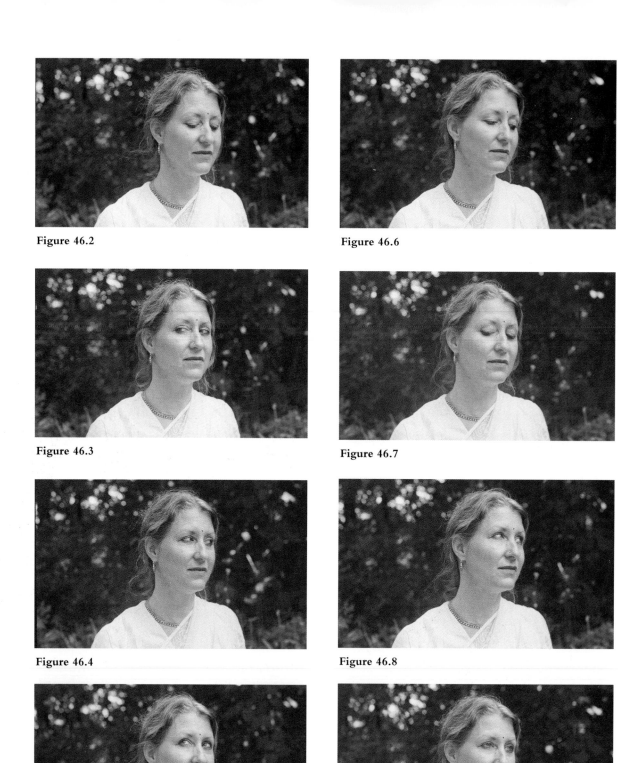

Figure 46.2

Figure 46.6

Figure 46.3

Figure 46.7

Figure 46.4

Figure 46.8

Figure 46.5

Figure 46.9

Next, look down (fig. 46.2). Moving your eyes slowly, look to the right (fig. 46.3). Next, look to the left (fig. 46.4). Now look to the upper right (fig. 46.5). Then look to the lower left (fig. 46.6). Look to the lower right (fig. 46.7). And look to the upper left (fig. 46.8). Finally, finish by looking to the front (fig. 46.9).

Now imagine a clock with numbers on it. Move your eyes very slowly in a clockwise direction through all the numbers, then reverse the order and move your eyes in a counterclockwise direction, "looking" at each number as you go.

Key: Do not strain your eyes, but do move them deliberately and, as much as possible, without blinking.

Benefits: This asana reduces eye strain and maintains neurological pathways from the eyes to the brain.

Neck Stretch

Sit in a cross-legged position with your back straight (fig. 47.1). Inhale and, without moving your shoul-

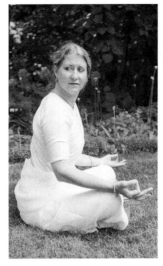

Figure 47.2

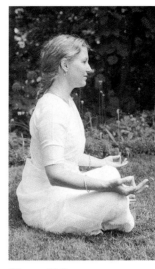

Figure 47.3

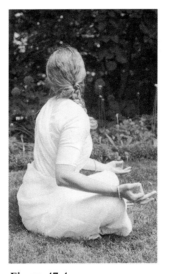

Figure 47.4

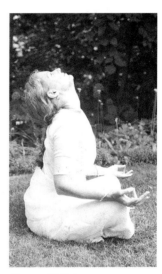

Figure 47.5

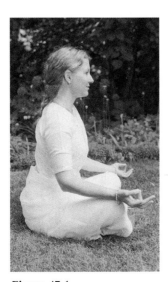

Figure 47.1

ders, turn your head slowly to the right and look as far right as possible (fig. 47.2). Exhale and turn your face to the front (fig. 47.3). Inhale, turning your head to the far left (fig. 47.4). Again, slowly exhale front.

Inhale and, while using maximum control over your neck muscles, extend your head as far back as possible (fig. 47.5). On exhale, lower your head as far forward as you can so that, if possible, your chin is touching your chest (fig. 47.6). Inhale and very slowly and consciously roll your head to the right (fig. 47.7). Still inhaling, roll your head past your

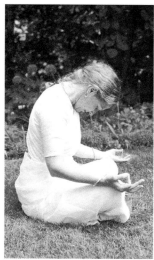
Figure 47.6

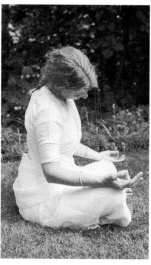
Figure 47.7

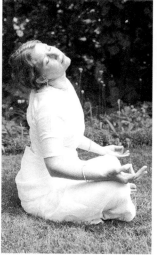
Figure 47.8

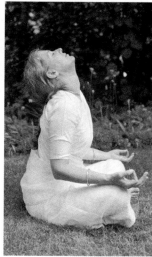
Figure 47.9

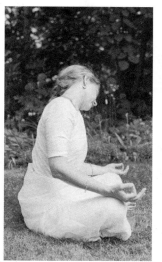
Figure 47.10

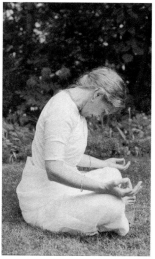
Figure 47.11

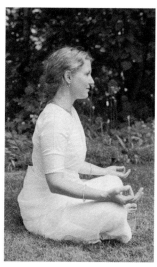
Figure 47.12

right shoulder and all the way around to the back, so that your head is resting backward on your upper back (figs. 47.8 and 47.9). Exhale and continue to roll your head around to the left, over your left shoulder and all the way to the front (figs. 47.10 and 47.11). On the inhale, raise your head to the central starting position (fig. 47.12).

Repeat the asana by reversing directions, beginning with turning your head to the left.

Key: At no point should you completely relax your neck muscles so that your head is just hanging on its own weight. It is important to visualize this as a stretching exercise so that you maintain control over your neck muscles at all times. This exercise should be done slowly and carefully. In the beginning you may not have full range of motion in your neck, but you can slowly work up to it.

Benefits: This asana develops strong and flexible neck muscles, which help reduce tension in the neck and shoulders.

Between Heaven and Earth: Asanas of Balance

(Element: Space)

Balance is a major part of yoga and one of the most essential elements of dance. In the following asanas we balance between heaven and earth, our bodies filling the space and mediating between the groundedness of earth and the transcendence of sky. Moving between the two, conscious repetition leads to grace on all levels.

In the next two asanas, begin by centering your concentration on the third, or womb, chakra, just below the navel. Then practice moving the center of your awareness, extending it from the womb to the lowest (muladhara) chakra at the base of the spine, then back to the womb center, and then upward to the highest chakra in the top of the head.

The Cat

Begin on all fours, kneeling on your hands and knees (fig. 48.1). On an inhale, expand your abdomen and lungs, raising your head to look skyward while dropping your lower back into a concave position (fig. 48.2). Exhale and contract your

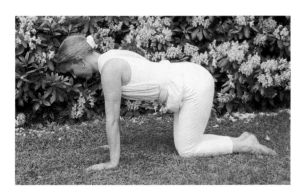

Figure 48.1

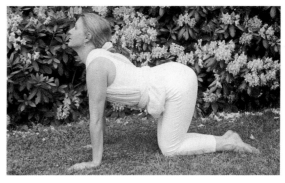

Figure 48.2

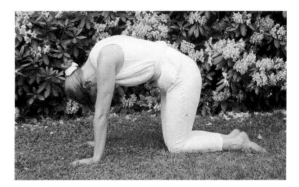

Figure 48.3

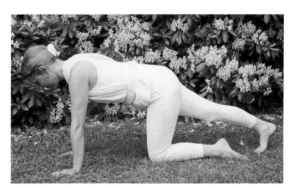

Figure 48.4

abdominal muscles, drawing them up toward your spine while dropping your head down between your elbows and simultaneously raising your back into a convex position (fig. 48.3). Repeat slowly three times.

On the next exhalation extend your right leg straight back, your right foot in a flexed position (fig. 48.4). Inhale and exhale, lowering and lifting

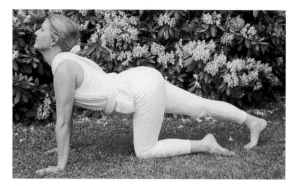

Figure 48.5

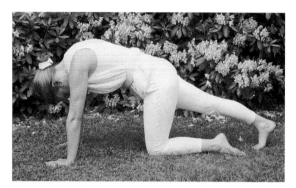

Figure 48.6

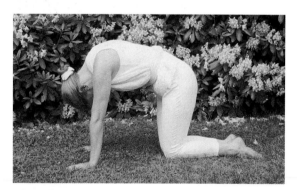

Figure 48.7

the spine and head, keeping the leg extended backward (figs. 48.5 and 48.6). Repeat three times on each side. On the final exhale, bring the extended leg back to its starting position, curving your back upward for a final stretch (fig. 48.7).

Key: When you exhale it is good to lift your back as high as possible. However, do not strain your back by forcing it too far into the concave position on the inhale.

Benefits: The cat is one of the simplest asanas for stretching the spine, while the one-leg variation also keeps the tendons in the back of your legs flexible.

The Flying Cat

For this next variation on the Cat pose, begin as in the previous asana by lifting your head and expanding your lungs on the inhalation (fig. 49.1). On the exhale extend your left arm forward and your right leg back, your head facing down (fig. 49.2).

Now inhale and stretch upward, lifting your head, arm, and leg (fig. 49.3). Exhale and reach

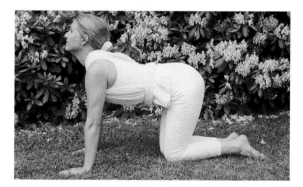

Figure 49.1

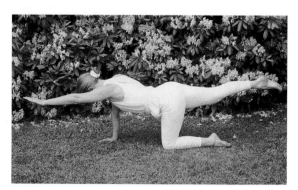

Figure 49.2

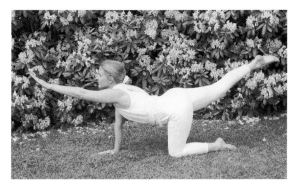

Figure 49.3

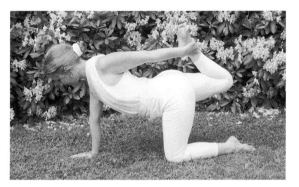

Figure 49.4

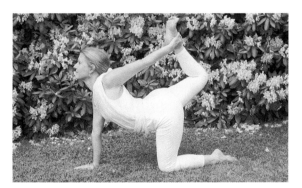

Figure 49.5

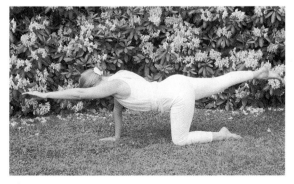

Figure 49.6

back with your left arm to grasp your right ankle (fig. 49.4). Inhale and pull up on your leg, stretching out and up as much as possible (fig. 49.5). On exhale, release your leg and straighten both arm and leg out once more (fig. 49.6).

Inhale and stretch outward and upward one more time (fig. 49.7). Hold this position as long as you can. Exhale and lower both arm and leg, raising your spine to make a convex curve (fig. 49.8).

Repeat the asana on the other side, extending your right arm and left leg. To complete the entire asana sequence, inhale and raise your head as in the first position of the Cat (fig. 49.9). On exhale, bring your right knee forward and lower your head until your knee touches your nose (fig. 49.10). Inhale and lift your leg as high up behind you as possible, stretching your lower back muscles and at the same time lifting your chin and looking up

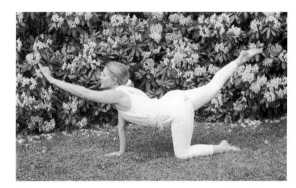

Figure 49.7

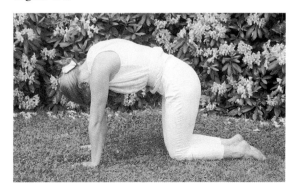

Figure 49.8

THE DANCE OF YOGA ❈ 133

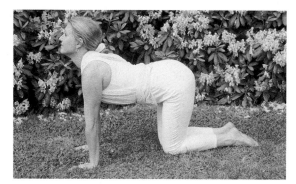

Figure 49.9

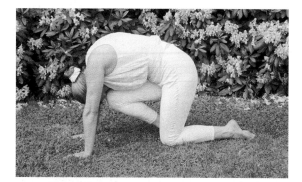

Figure 49.10

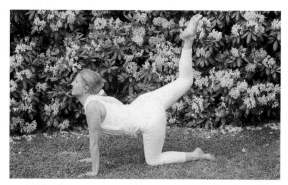

Figure 49.11

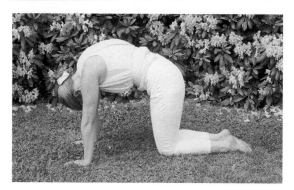

Figure 49.12

(fig. 49.11). Hold this position and breathe for one round. On exhale, lower your leg and raise your back for a counter-stretch (fig. 49.12).

Repeat this final sequence on the other side to end.

Key: Whenever shifting from the concave to the convex position, begin the movement by raising the middle of your back straight up and letting your neck, head, and eyes follow. On the exhalations be sure to work your abdominal muscles by pulling your navel inward toward your spine.

Benefits: While strengthening upper arms and lower back, this asana also promotes balance.

The Shoulderstand is extremely beneficial for circulation, as the heart works against gravity to supply blood to the inverted extremities. Here I add dynamism to this standard asana by combining it with leg movements that end in the Bridge, my favorite pelvic stretch.

Shoulderstand with Pelvis Stretch

Begin by lying on the earth with your knees bent, your thighs against your chest, and your hands placed under your lower back, palms up (fig. 50.1). Using your hands to assist you, roll through your torso until your thighs are parallel to the earth (fig. 50.2). Inhale and exhale in place. Now, on exhale, straighten your legs so that they are parallel to the ground, feet extended behind you (fig. 50.3). Hold and breathe.

Raise your legs, keeping your back as straight as possible (fig. 50.4). Bend at the neck and shoulders, not the middle of your back. Hold this position and breathe, expanding and contracting your abdomen.

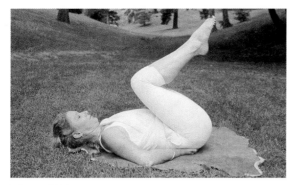

Figure 50.1

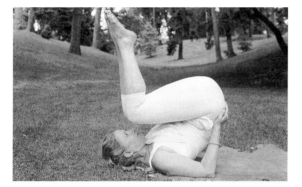

Figure 50.2

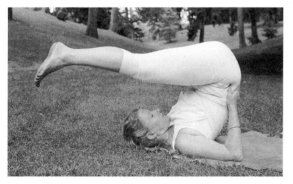

Figure 50.3

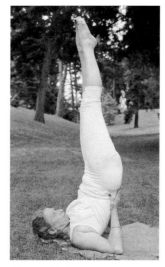

Figure 50.4

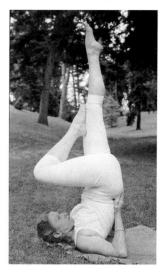

Figure 50.5

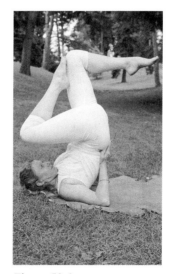

Figure 50.6

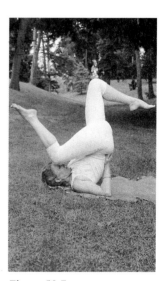

Figure 50.7

On an exhale, bend your right knee so that your right foot touches your left knee and your right thigh is parallel to the earth (fig. 50.5). Hold and breathe. On an exhale, still keeping your back straight, bend your left leg at the knee, so that your left lower leg is perpendicular to your left thigh (fig. 50.6).

As you exhale, begin to lower your spine toward the earth, extending your left foot downward toward the earth and your right knee backward toward your chest (fig. 50.7). Stretch slowly downward until the ball of your left foot touches the ground, then rest your right foot on your left knee (fig. 50.8). Hold and breathe, expanding your abdomen on the inhale.

On an exhale bring your right foot down to the ground next to your left foot (fig. 50.9). Hold and breathe, expanding on the inhale and contracting on the exhale. To finish, on an exhale slowly lower your spine to starting postion (fig. 50.10).

THE DANCE OF YOGA ❊ 135

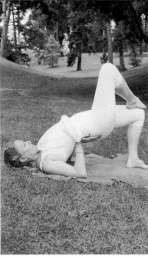
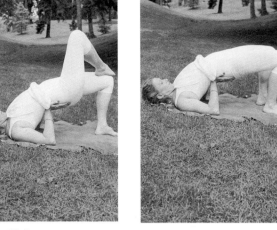

Figure 50.8 **Figure 50.9**

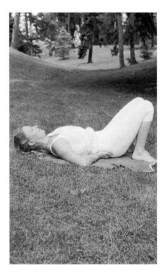

Figure 50.10

Repeat the entire sequence leading with your right foot.

Key: Be sure to perform this asana on a soft mat or cushion in order not to injure the bones in your neck. After completing the series, breathe in a relaxed position before sitting up.

Benefits: This asana promotes flexibility of the spine andeases blood circulation in the face and the glands located in the neck and upper thorax.

The Headstand is one of the most popular of all yoga asanas. It is a radically effective way to increase blood flow to the brain and to the glands in the upper body; it also promotes balance and strengthens the lower back. It is one of the few asanas that directly impacts the crown chakra at the top of the skull, as well as the ajna chakra, or "third eye," located at the pineal gland. For this reason the Headstand should be practiced carefully. If done correctly, it can be a lot of fun—the Headstand turns the world upside down and gives you a different perspective on the gravity of life. Instead of thinking that I am standing on my head, I like to think that I am standing on the sky, holding up the earth.

The Headstand

Begin by sitting on your knees on a cushion or folded blanket (fig. 51.1). Bending your arms, lean forward and place your hands such that your head and arms form a triangular base (fig. 51.2). Walk forward (fig. 51.3) close enough to your arms that

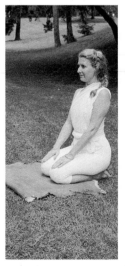 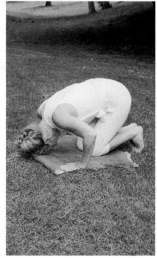

Figure 51.1 **Figure 51.2**

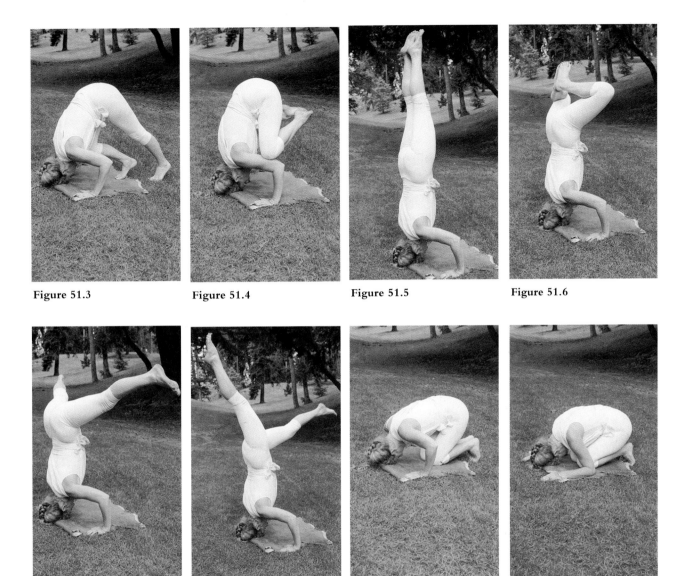

Figure 51.3 Figure 51.4 Figure 51.5 Figure 51.6

Figure 51.7 Figure 51.8 Figure 51.9 Figure 51.10

you can lift one leg, then the other, up onto your arms (fig. 51.4). Hold this position and breathe until you feel steady and balanced.

Using the muscles of your lower back to control your movements, slowly straighten one leg, then the other, above your head (fig. 51.5). When you are balanced, practice deep breathing, expanding on the inhalation and contracting on the exhalation.

Now try the following variations. Open your legs and join the soles of your feet (fig. 51.6).

Spread your legs out to the side as far as they can go (fig. 51.7). Spread your legs forward and backward into a scissors position (fig. 51.8).

Finally, return to the straight-leg position. Bending your knees, lower your legs to the earth once more (fig. 51.9). Bring your arms down to rest on the earth (fig. 51.10). Rest in this position for a few moments, keeping your head on the ground. Slowly return to an upright, seated position.

Key: Use the muscles of your lower back to steady

THE DANCE OF YOGA ❧ 137

yourself and maintain balance. Do not remain in the Headstand for more than a few minutes, especially if you feel pressure behind your eyes.

Benefits: This asana increases blood circulation to the region of the brain and face. It promotes balance and, like the Shoulderstand, develops strength in the lower back.

The swastik is an ancient fertility symbol found everywhere in Indian culture. For thousands of years it has been associated in India with the worship of the sun. It also stands for shakti, energy and power, the feminine creative principle. In this asana the body becomes a swastik in order to invoke this same sense of power and energy within. Keep concentration centered on the womb center, the third or manipura chakra.

The Swastik

Start in a basic standing position, your legs together, back straight, and hands at your sides (fig. 52.1). Inhale and raise your hands, placing

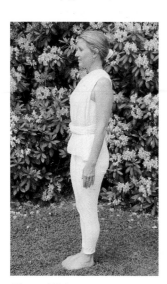

Figure 52.1

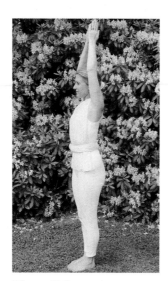

Figure 52.2

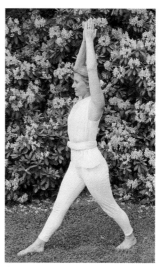

Figure 52.3

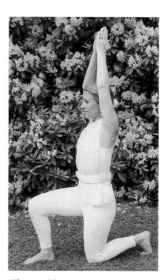

Figure 52.4

your palms together over your head (fig. 52.2). On the exhale, step forward with your right leg, standing with both your front and back legs straight (fig. 52.3). Inhale in place.

Exhale and bend both your knees so that your right thigh is parallel to the ground and your left knee is resting on the ground, both legs forming right angles (fig. 52.4). Inhale in position, stretching your spine and flattening your back by keeping your pelvis tilted slightly forward. On exhale, turn your upper body to the right. With your hands in

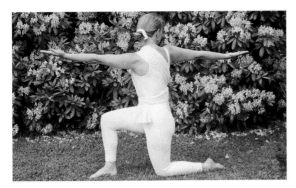

Figure 52.5

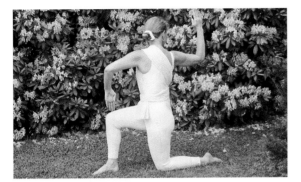

Figure 52.6

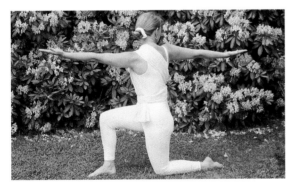

Figure 52.7

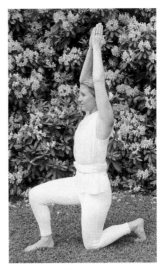

Figure 52.8

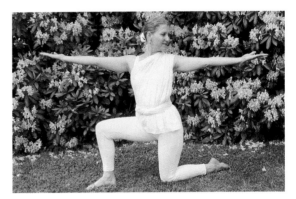

Figure 52.9

pataka mudra, lower your arms until they are in a straight line with your shoulders and aligned with your legs, holding both your right and left palms up (fig. 52.5). Inhale and exhale in place, looking back at your right hand.

Inhale and bend both your elbows so that your right hand is raised up, palm facing front, and your left upper arm is lowered, palm facing back (fig. 52.6). Your arms and legs should both form right angles. Inhale and exhale in place. Inhale again and, on exhale, straighten your arms to the former position (fig. 52.7). Inhale and exhale in place. Inhale once more. On exhale turn to the front, raising your hands over your head (fig. 52.8). Inhale in place.

Exhale and turn this time to the left, opening your arms out so that both palms are facing upward (fig. 52.9). Look at your left hand. Inhale in place. Exhale and bend your elbows so that your left forearm is raised up, palm facing front, and your right forearm faces down, palm facing back (fig. 52.10). Inhale and exhale in place. Inhale and turn to the front again, raising your hands over your head (fig. 52.11).

THE DANCE OF YOGA ❦ 139

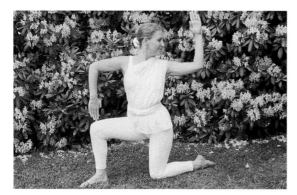

Figure 52.10

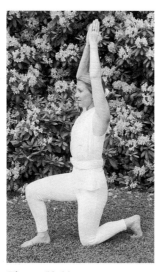

Figure 52.11

To return to standing position, inhale. On exhale, shift your weight onto your right leg and stand up, bringing your left leg forward.

Key: To create the ideal form (based on right angles), visualize how your body looks from the outside.

Benefits: This asana stretches your arms, shoulders, and waist, and develops a keen sense of balance.

※

This asana is quite demanding. An excellent preparation for Indian dance, it develops strength in the legs and the lower back as well as a more commanding sense of balance. Keeping concentration at the third chakra assists your balance by establishing a pivotal point in the body close to the earth.

The Solid Stretch

Begin by leaning on your left knee, your right knee bent and your right foot on the ground, both legs forming right angles. Join your palms in front of your chest, elbows up (fig. 53.1). On exhale, lower your arms and place your hands on the ground on either side of your right foot, leaning your upper body forward so that your chest is held against your right leg (fig. 53.2). Inhale in place.

Keeping both feet in place and your right thigh parallel to the ground, straighten your back leg on the exhalation (fig. 53.3). Inhale and straighten and lift your back until you are sitting up, your palms joined in front of your chest (fig. 53.4). Exhale in place.

Inhale and lift your arms over your head, stretching up and back (fig. 53.5). Exhale and lean your upper body all the way forward so that your upper body is stretched out over your right bent knee, your spine as straight as possible (fig. 53.6). Inhale

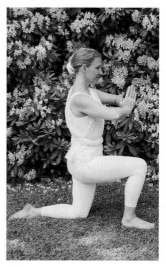

Figure 53.1

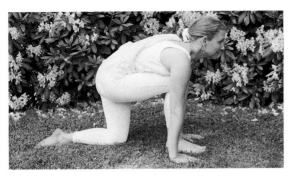

Figure 53.2

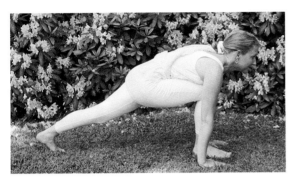

Figure 53.3

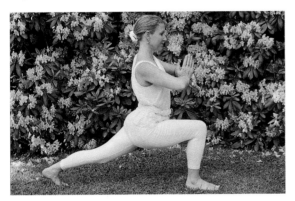

Figure 53.4

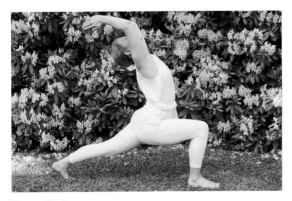

Figure 53.5

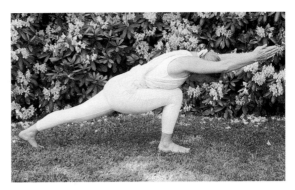

Figure 53.6

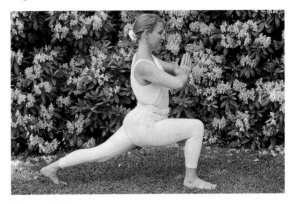

Figure 53.7

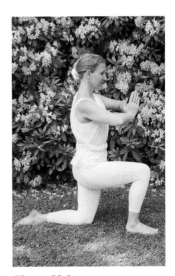

Figure 53.8

and pull up into the sitting position, palms in front of your chest (fig. 53.7). Exhale and slowly lower your left knee (fig. 53.8). Inhale in place. On exhale, return to a standing position. Inhale and lean on your right knee to begin the asana on the other side.

Key: Once they are in position, hold your legs as firmly as possible so that only your upper body is moving. Use control to lower your knee to the floor.

Benefits: This asana develops tremendous strength in your thighs, and stretches your leg muscles and your entire spine. It also helps to develop balance.

❧

Because the following three asanas involve standing on one leg, it becomes very important to find your body's pivotal center of balance at the beginning of each sequence. You will find it somewhere around the third, or manipura, chakra, a few inches beneath the navel. Think in terms of establishing your center close to the ground by sinking into the lower part of your body before you attempt to move any other part of your body. Retain control over your balance by remembering not to lock the knee of the leg on which you are standing.

The One-Leg Standing Stretch

Standing on your left leg, lift your right knee up to your chest and grasp your ankle with both hands

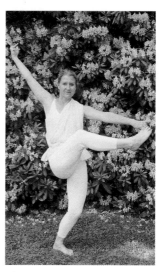

Figure 54.3

(fig. 54.1). Hold this position and inhale. On the next exhalation, raise your right arm straight over your head in alapadma mudra while you continue to grasp your right ankle with your right hand (fig. 54.2). Try to keep your trunk straight. Hold and breathe one round.

On the next exhalation, stretch your right leg across your body and your right arm to the right at a forty-five-degree angle (fig. 54.3). Hold and breathe. Release your ankle on an exhale and slowly lower your leg to the floor.

Repeat the sequence on the other side.

Key: Slightly bend the knee of the leg you are standing on to retain control over your balance. Hold your lower back and abdominal muscles tight, even as you lift your leg.

Benefits: This asana stretches your thigh muscles and develops balance and strength.

The Dancer's Front Bend

Standing on your left leg with your right leg bent, clasp your right ankle with your right hand, and raise your left arm directly overhead (fig. 55.1). Making your back as straight as possible, inhale in

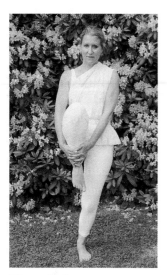

Figure 54.1

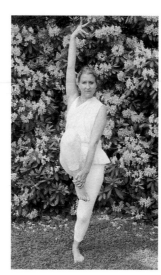

Figure 54.2

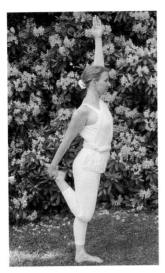

Figure 55.1

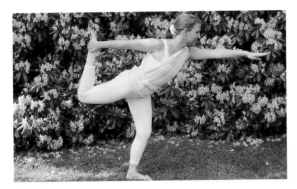

Figure 55.2

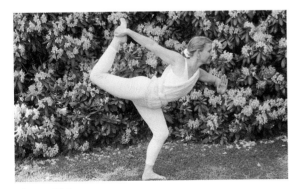

Figure 55.3

than your foot. Bend your left arm and bring your palm in front of your chest to complete the pose (fig. 55.3). Exhale in place. Inhale once more and, on exhale, slowly lower your raised leg as you return to a standing position.

Key: Control your leg muscles by contracting them. To help your balance, maintain your center of gravity while leaning forward.

Benefits: This asana stretches your spine and arm and leg muscles as it develops balance.

This asana replicates the sculpted images of dancers that adorn the walls of temples throughout India. To complete the effect, be sure to look down at your lower hand as you lean into the pose.

The Dancer's Side Bend

Standing on your left leg, raise your right knee up in front of you so that your pointed toe is held at the level of your knee. Rest both palms on your lifted knee (fig. 56.1). Inhale in place. On exhale

place. On exhale, lean forward and extend your left arm in front of you while pulling your right leg upward (fig. 55.2). Inhale and exhale in place.

On the next inhale, raise your right leg as high as possible behind you so that your head is lower

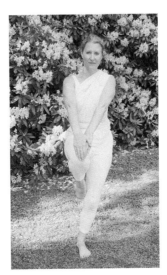

Figure 56.1

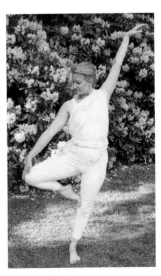

Figure 56.2

THE DANCE OF YOGA ❦ 143

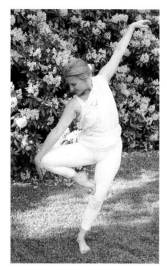
Figure 56.3

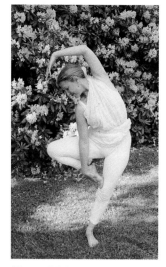
Figure 56.4

Benefits: This asana stretches the upper body as it develops balance.

Natraj (Dancing Shiva)

Standing in a bent-knee position, your toes turned out to the side, raise your left leg across the front of your body. Your right hand is in pataka mudra, with your palm facing front. Your left hand is extended across your body in line with the raised leg, and the left hand hangs gracefully from the wrist. Be sure to keep your elbows lifted (fig. 57). Hold this position and breathe.

Reverse sides to execute the same asana.

open your right knee out to the right, keeping your right hand on your knee and raising your left arm up and out to the left at a forty-five-degree angle (fig. 56.2). Inhale and stretch your spine upward.

On exhale, shift your weight toward the right and bend your upper body slightly toward the right (fig. 56.3). Inhale in place. Finally, on exhale, lean farther toward your raised leg, fully bending sideways at the waist and reaching down with your right hand to touch your right foot. Bend your left arm and reach over the top of your head with your left hand (fig. 56.4). Inhale and exhale in place.

Repeat the entire sequence, this time standing on your right leg and clasping your left ankle with your left hand.

Now perform the same sequence in a reverse direction, moving back through each position, taking time to breathe in each position and moving on the exhalations.

Repeat on the other side, beginning with raising the left leg.

Key: Get a firm footing by finding your center of balance and by firmly controlling your lower back and abdominal muscles.

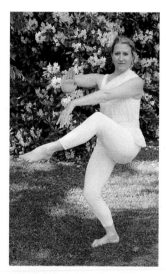
Figure 57

Key: To maintain your balance, you must keep the leg on which you are standing bent as much as possible. Face front while extending the left arm and leg across your body.

Benefits: This asana strengthens the muscles of both arms and legs and promotes balance.

The undisputed king of modern hatha yoga, Surya Namaskar was created nearly a hundred years ago by the maharaja of Oundh, a small kingdom in the western state of Maharastra. Using Vedic sun invocations as his model, the maharaja's intention was to combine the meditative quality of traditional prayer with an athletic yoga exercise that would keep the body fit. The result is an asana that, appealing to both East and West, is now practiced throughout the world. While several variations on Surya Namaskar have been developed, the following is the original version developed by the maharaja. It was taught to me by his son, Sri Apa Pant.

Surya Namaskar (Salute to the Sun)

Stand facing the sun, your back straight, palms joined in front of your chest (fig. 58.1). Inhale, raising your arms over your head and stretching up and back (fig. 58.2). Exhale and lower your arms to the ground, placing your hands beside your feet and bringing your head to your knees (fig. 58.3).

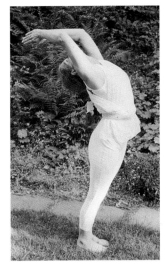

Figure 58.2

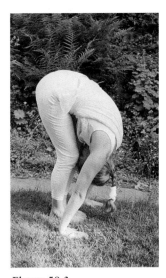

Figure 58.3

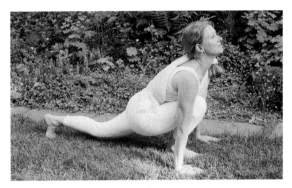

Figure 58.4

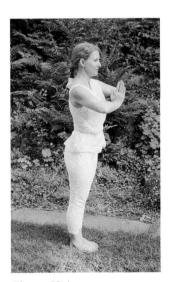

Figure 58.1

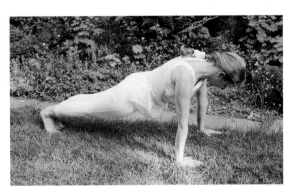

Figure 58.5

Try to keep your legs as straight as possible.

Inhale and, keeping your palms on the earth, extend your left leg back and look up (fig. 58.4). Holding your breath, put your weight on your arms and extend your right leg behind you (fig. 58.5).

THE DANCE OF YOGA ❈ 145

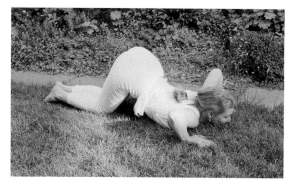

Figure 58.6

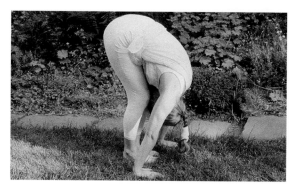

Figure 58.10

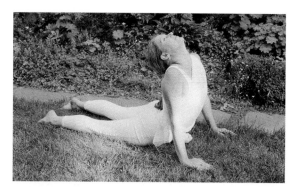

Figure 58.7

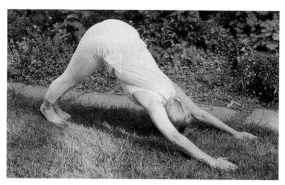

Figure 58.8

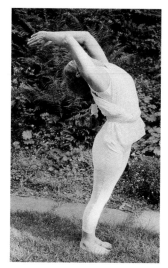

Figure 58.11

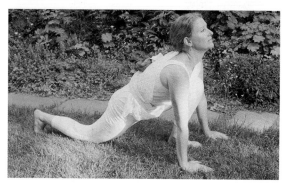

Figure 58.9

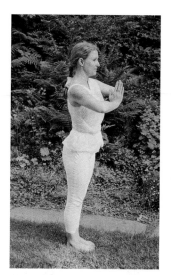

Figure 58.12

Keep your back straight as you balance on your hands and feet.

Exhale and, shifting your weight slowly forward, keep moving until your knees, chest, and chin are on the ground, your lower back in a radically concave position (fig. 58.6). Inhale and push forward and up into a full Cobra position, your pelvis on the ground and your neck extended backward as you look up (fig. 58.7). Exhale, lifting your body up onto your arms and legs, lowering your head between your extended arms and pushing back (fig. 58.8). Keep your legs straight so that you feel the pull in the tendons in the back of your legs.

Inhale, bringing your left knee forward into a bent position and raising your chin to look up (fig. 58.9). Exhale, bringing your back leg forward and lowering your head to your knees (fig. 58.10). Inhale and stretch up and back (fig. 58.11). Finish by standing up, bringing your palms together in front of your chest (fig. 58.12).

Repeat the entire sequence, this time extending your right leg backward. Alternate sides until you have performed a total of twelve Surya Namaskars.

Key: This asana may be performed slowly to relax you, or with vigor to wake you up. The fifth and sixth positions are the ones people most often find difficult. In the fifth position, it is important to keep your back flat and straight. In the sixth position, make sure that you move far enough forward so that you do not strain your lower back. Keep moving forward until your chest is nearly even with your hands.

Benefits: This series offers an excellent overall stretch, a workout for the lungs, and a balanced movement that in itself resembles a dance. I cannot recommend it highly enough.

Meditative Postures: Going Within
(Elements: Earth, Water, Fire, Air, and Space)

While all of the asanas thus far have been dynamic exercises, designed to flow into one another, there is also a time to stop action in order to go deeper within one's consciousness. The following asanas are my favorites for this purpose. They represent different attitudes of mind and body for actively seeking inner peace and calm.

Classic Meditation Posture

This is also known as the modified *padmasan* pose. Sitting cross-legged on the ground with a straight spine, level shoulders, and expanded chest, gracefully rest your hands on your knees, your hands in arala mudra (fig. 59). Focus your closed eyes in the space between your eyebrows. Keeping a slight smile on your lips, breathe deeply.

I use this posture to open myself to my surroundings and imagine dissolving my limited self in nature and the cosmos.

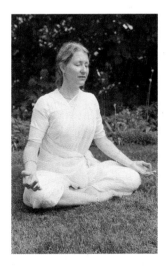

Figure 59

Zen Posture

Sitting on your knees for any length of time requires tremendous discipline and the ability to ignore your legs when they fall asleep. But sometimes for shorter periods of meditation or for intense focus, I prefer this self-contained posture (fig. 60). It allows me to withdraw within rather than expand outward. This position is excellent for abiding in the moment, simply being rather than doing anything at all.

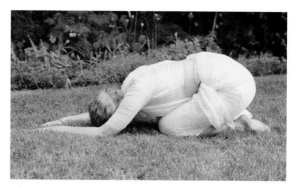

Figure 61

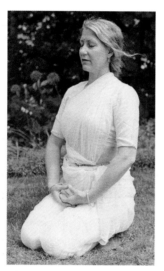

Figure 60

Resting on the Earth

From sitting on your knees in the Zen Posture, extend your arms forward until your forehead is resting on the ground (fig. 61). With open palms and forearms facing downward, relax your spine as your buttocks rest on your calves.

In this position I slowly inhale and exhale, taking in the prana or life force of Mother Earth as I smell the grass and dampness of Earth and take refuge in her dark solidity. I find this both a restful and incredibly consoling way to recharge myself when I am stressed.

Child of the Earth

From the position of Resting on the Earth, turn your head to either side and bring your arms back so that they are resting alongside your body (fig. 62). Breathe deeply.

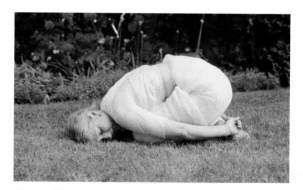

Figure 62

This is known as the child's pose for a very good reason. By contracting into a near-fetal position you draw all your energy inward and protect the third chakra area, the center of will. This is a comfortable way to restore your energy while feeling the connection to Mother Earth. Warning: If you are not careful, you will soon be asleep!

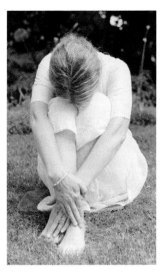

Figure 63

Time Out

This posture is another way of withdrawing into the self. When you are feeling sad or overwhelmed, this body language speaks of the need to be left alone for a time so that damaged parts of the self have a chance to heal. Lean forward and literally block out all light by placing your eyes against your knees (fig. 63). Breathe deeply and give yourself calming suggestions to soothe stress and tensions.

I usually follow a few moments of this posture with a straight-backed basic posture that says I am ready to face the world again.

Yoganidra (Sleeping Yoga)

Lie flat on your back, eyes closed and muscles completely relaxed (fig. 64). Focus on your breathing. From this position it is easy to enter a type of sleep in which you retain a part of your waking consciousness as you begin to slide into the dreamworld. Conscious dreaming begins with a kind of free-floating association of images, and resembles the state we first enter as we fall asleep. The difference is in the ability to remain conscious, which comes only with practice.

The Yoganidra posture allows us to explore the terrain not only between the wakeful and dreaming states but between life and death as well. Yogis in India sometimes meditate in this way in order to reconcile themselves to their own mortality. Not coincidentally, this is also the posture most conducive to out-of-body, or astral, traveling.

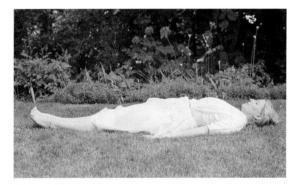

Figure 64

FIVE

Yoga of the Emotions
Spiritual Dimensions of Indian Drama

The practical applications of this yoga of Indian dance about which you are reading involve not only the physical body but the mind and emotions as well. The authoritative text governing all aspects of dance and drama, the *Natya Sastra,* offers great insight into human psychology in typically Indian fashion: through a system that classifies human emotion into nine main rasas, "essences" or "flavors." These are *sringara* (the erotic), *hasya* (the humorous), *karuna* (the compassionate), *raudra* (the fierce), *vira* (the heroic), *bhayanaka* (the fearful), *bibatsa* (the disgusted), *adbhuta* (the wondrous), and *santa* (the peaceful). Later texts and traditions enumerate even more rasas, but these nine are the rasas most generally recognized.

According to Indian aesthetics, the term *rasa* technically refers to the experience invoked by drama in the audience or witness, the *rasika* ("taster" or "enjoyer"), while the actual feelings or emotions portrayed by the dancer are referred to as *bhavas*. The rasika, or audience member, is as important to the success of a dramatic undertaking as the performer, for without someone to witness, even the best artistic production is wasted. Therefore the *Natya Sastra* lists the qualifications not only for performers but for audiences as well. Different forms of art exist for different audiences.

Bhavas are further classified in aesthetic theory as permanent, fleeting, or innate. Each rasa or archetypal essence has particular bhavas associated with it, and these emotions color the archetype in particular ways. When portraying a particular character in a drama, the predominant rasa or rasas associated with that character would be prescribed in advance, and it was up to the artist to stay within these parameters set by the tradition. Of course, there was much

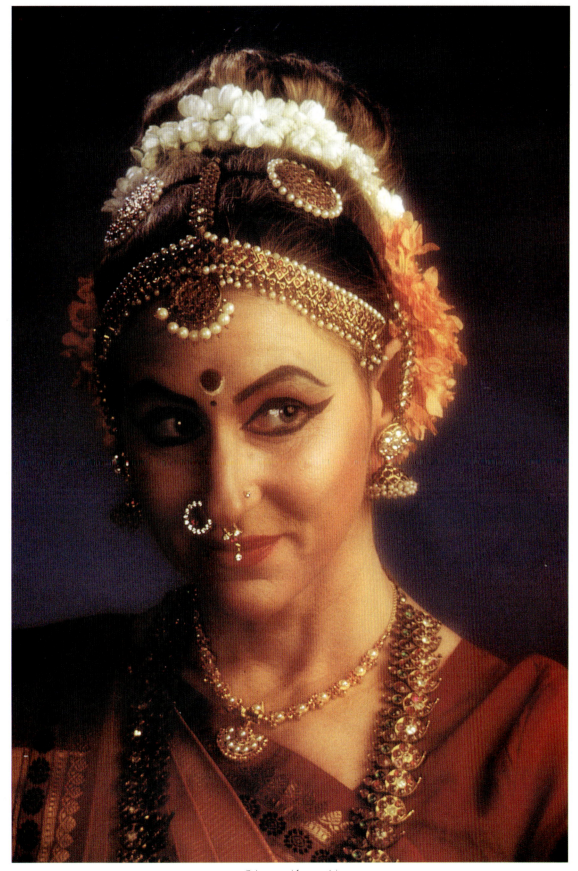
Sringara (the erotic)

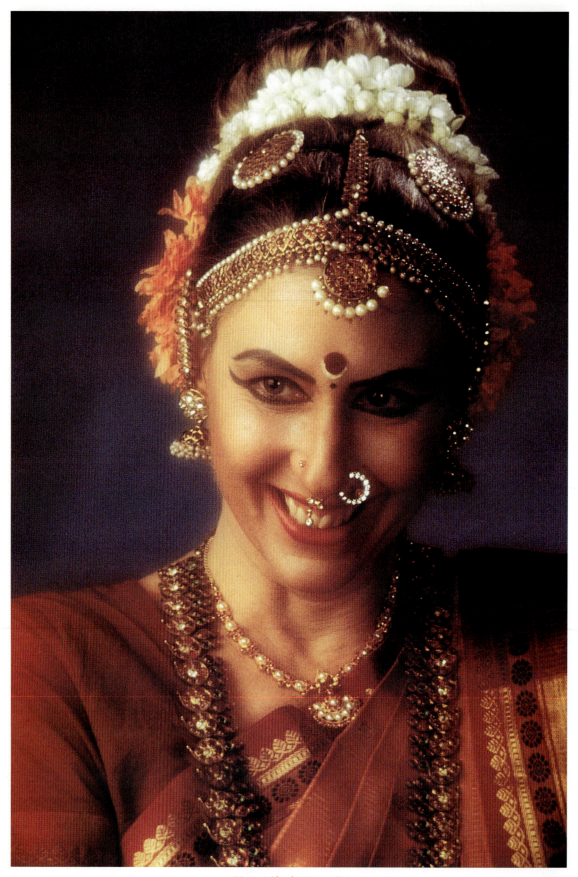
Hasya (the humorous)

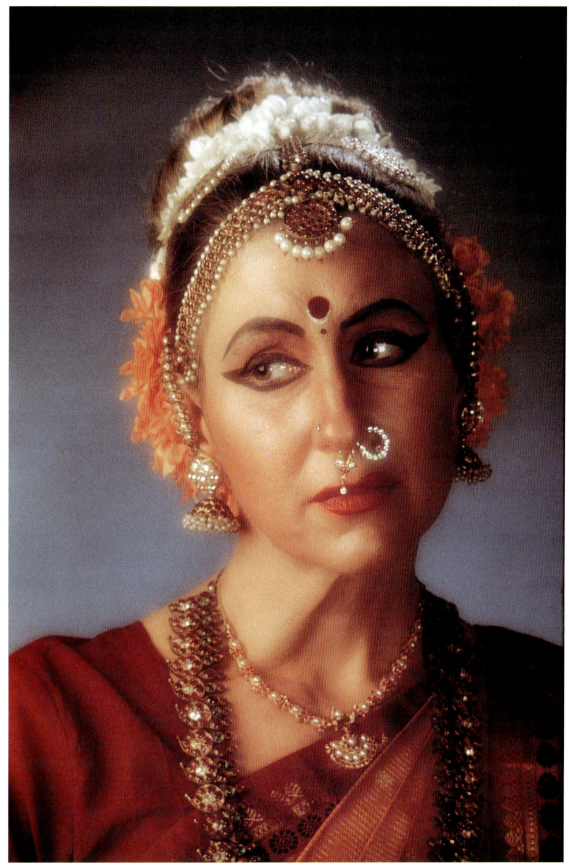
Karuna (the compassionate)

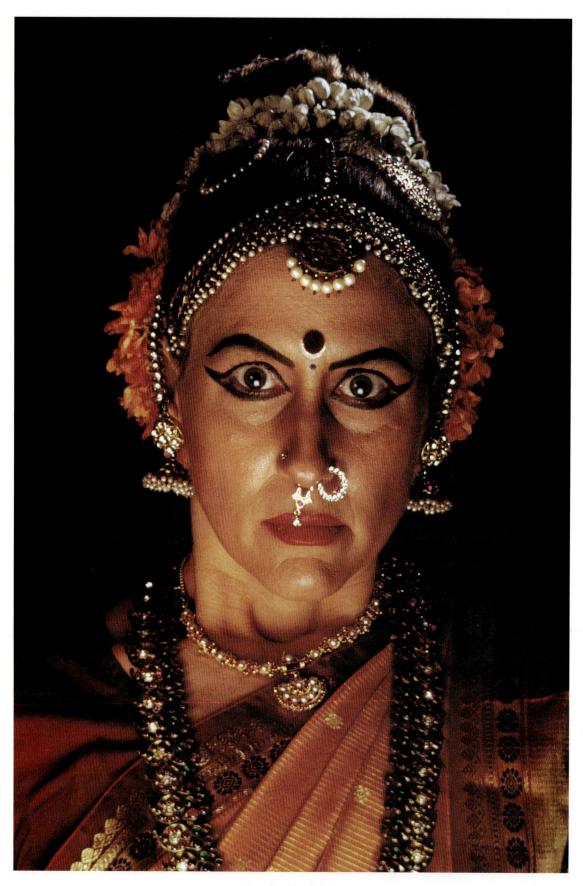
Raudra (the fierce)

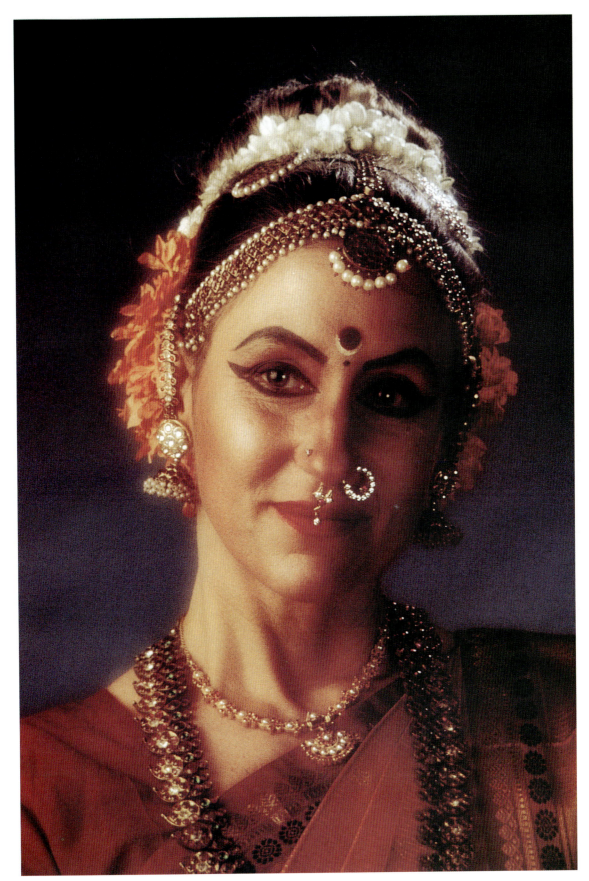

Vira (the heroic)

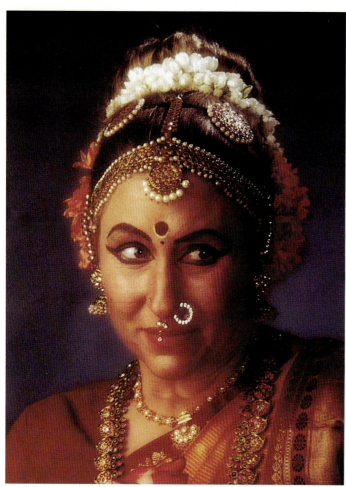

Bhayanaka (the fearful)

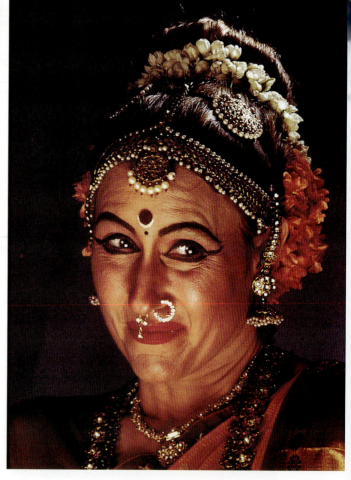

Bibatsa (the disgusted)

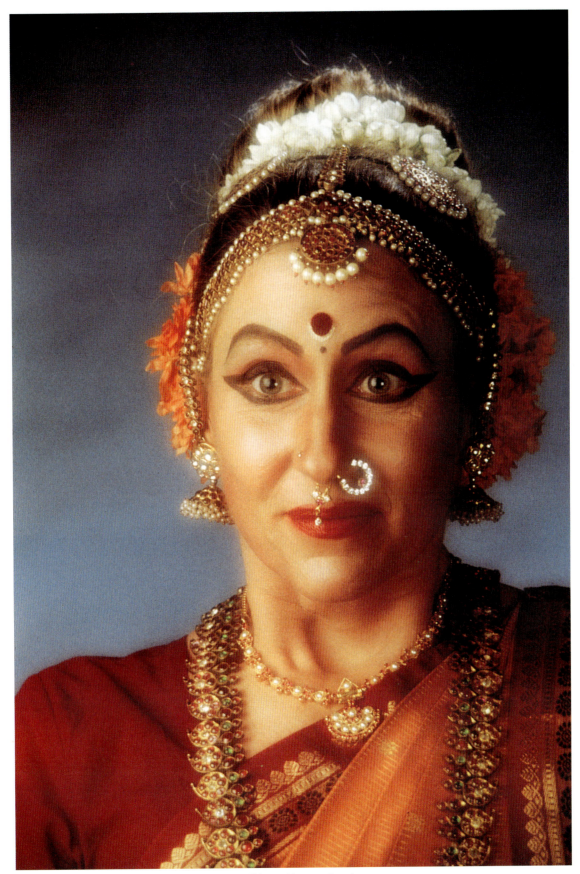
Adbhuta (the wondrous)

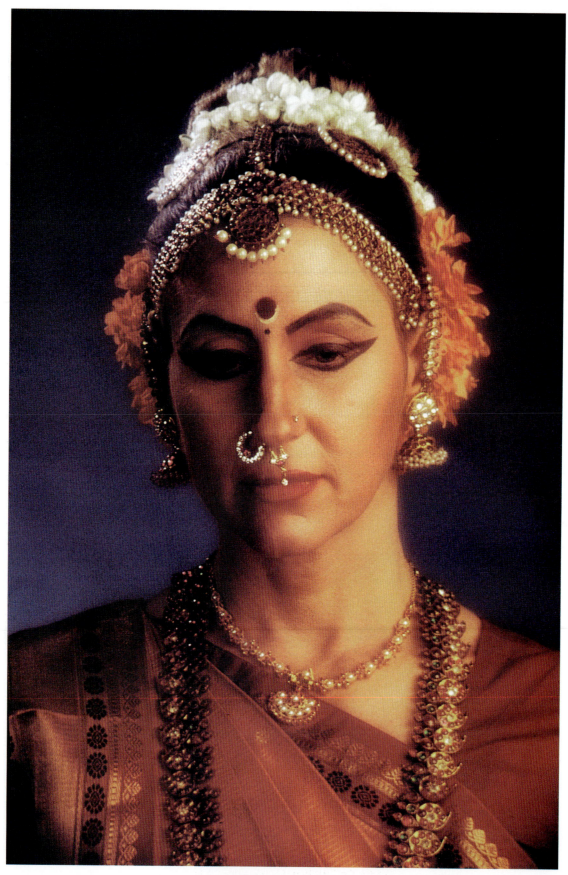

Santa (the peaceful)

discussion and debate within the culture regarding the nature of rasa and bhava, as evidenced by the existence of several treatises and commentaries on the subject of Indian aesthetics.

One of those debates was over which rasa was superior to all others. In most dance and drama it is undoubtedly sringara, the erotic, which predominates. Perhaps this is because from the beginning Hindus have recognized that eros, desire, is at the root of creation. It is how we got here, and why we hate to leave our bodies. It is the source of all attachment, bringing the greatest joy and also the greatest sorrow. In the drama of life itself, eros predominates.

The Hindu understanding and acceptance of desire is one of the most profound aspects of its spiritual teachings. This marks the major difference between the religious art forms of East and West. In India there is no distinction between the sacred and the erotic. Whether in painting, sculpture, poetry, or dance, erotic desire is not only permissible, it is actually the preferred metaphor for expressing the longing of the human soul for the transcendent. Within the Hindu tradition there is no such thing as the kind of puritanism we in the West take for granted: one that equates purity with sexual abstinence and opposes the spirit to the body. Gods and goddesses, as well as humans, saints, and sages, are sexual beings with desire for each other and for the beauty of the world. Within both Hinduism and Buddhism, desire is recognized as a primary distinguishing characteristic of the human reality. As spiritual disciplines both religions work (albeit in different ways) to harness this desire toward higher ends.

Hinduism uses drama as a means of celebrating eros even while reflecting on desire's fleeting and illusory nature. The many shades and nuances of sringara, the erotic sentiment, are depicted in the arts both visually (in sculpture and painting) and orally (in music and poetry). Yet it is dance and drama, the most complex and highly evolved art forms, that incorporate the visual and the oral and add to these the kinesthetic experience. All three dimensions are found in the four kinds of abhinaya, or means of expression, listed in the *Natya Sastra:* bodily stance and ornamentation correspond to the visual, speech and music to the oral, and the display of subtle emotion to the kinesthetic.

It might seem surprising to interpret satvika, the most subtle aspect of the dance and drama, as kinesthetic, but for me one of the greatest insights of the Indian aesthetic tradition is that art practiced as a spiritual discipline is grounded in the body. Therefore it is recognized that the rasas (archetypal states) can only be truly understood when they are portrayed in bhavas, or emotions. In other words, the rasas can be perceived only when they are given form, and for that the human body, for all its imperfections, is still the most perfect vehicle. When the dancer employs satvika abhinaya she actually feels the emotions she is portraying; they manifest as physical sensations. These feelings are then picked up and experienced by the audience in a kind of sympathetic resonance.

The manner in which this resonance occurs is comparable to the Hindu understanding of darshan. As discussed in chapter one, darshan is a kind of transfer of energy between a god or guru and a devotee, often understood as taking place through the eyes. It is the act of seeing and being seen by the Divine. What is not often understood is that this transfer is experienced as substantial; that is, some substance, however subtle, is being exchanged. This same logic feeds into the pervasive belief in Indian culture (and in most other traditional cultures as well) in *dristhi,* or the "evil eye." Dristhi is one of the main reasons Hindu women wear a red bindi in the middle of their foreheads. It is believed that if someone looks upon a woman (or anyone) with lust, envy, or any other excessive emotion, that negative energy will be conveyed to the person through the gaze and could result in bad luck or illness. The red vermillion mark on the forehead is believed to protect one from that ill fortune. On the other hand the positive energy of an image of god, a sacred site, or an enlightened being (a saint or guru) is also understood as a physical emanation, one that is believed to have the power to heal and even to offer those who come into proximity and resonance with it a taste of enlightenment. However, it would be a mistake to limit our understanding of darshan, and the artistic process, to the visual dimension only. All the senses are involved. In fact, when satvika abhinaya is really effective all the senses are included and transcended in a total experience—the rasa experience—one that unites the seer and the seen, the dancer and the audience, the human and the Divine.

The means to achieve that state is through the individual rasas. Sringara, the erotic, was particularly effective because of the many nuances with which it could be colored. Some of the forms of sringara commonly depicted include love in union (fulfillment), love in separation (longing), love in anger, and so on. In these scenarios it is almost always the case that the beloved or object of desire is the male god or hero, while the lover is female. This is in keeping with Hindu philosophical attitudes toward nature and sexuality, which view the feminine principle as active while the masculine principle is dominant but nonetheless passive. The possibilities for the interaction of male and female are endless; in earlier centuries, when the arts proliferated, the classification of these archetypal variations became as important as their enactment on the stage or their appearance on canvas or in literature. Debate and discussion of these erotic themes flourished, for in concentrating on woman's relationship to man, scholars were actually contemplating something much more encompassing: humankind's relationship to God.

These philosophic debates regarding the finer points of aesthetic theory were traditionally not the concern of performers. Such discussions were mainly the pastime of the educated literary elite, those who wrote the dramas and for whom plays and dance performances were produced. While sringara, or the erotic archetype, was predominant for centuries, a later, more pious development in the tradition argued that all rasas merge finally into santa, the peaceful. This understandable theological move is in keeping with a tradition that ostensibly values transcendent unity and the withdrawal of the senses over the painful and messy reality of the human experience. However, Kalidasa, India's greatest classical dramatist whose works explore the entire gamut of the human and the Divine, held a slightly different position. He argued that there is really only one rasa that underlies all the others and that is karuna, the compassionate.

To me this is the wisest position of all, for if indeed the ideal goal of all our striving is peace, it is nonetheless true that the everyday reality of life as we experience it lies in the many desires we harbor, whether they are fulfilled or frustrated. In recognition of this relative or aesthetic (rather than absolute) nature of truth, the wisest response is not condemnation of human desire but acceptance of its place in life and in ourselves. It is to this sense of truth that drama bears witness. Desire is not only the cause of all suffering, it is also the basis of all compassion. This is essentially the tantric perspective, which is implicitly shared by the greatest of India's artists and aestheticians. It is a path of self-awareness that leads through, not above and over, desire.

The Rasa Experience

While spirituality was always implied in the arts of India, approximately one thousand years ago the tradition began explicitly comparing the highest goals of art to the mystical states, such as those attained while seeking *samadhi,* the final goal of yoga. Drawing upon the earliest understandings of dramatic theory found in the *Natya Sastra,* the term *rasa* came to refer not only to the archetypal "flavors," as a group, but also to pure "essence," a transcendent and blissful aesthetic experience. The process by which one attains this pure rasa has been analyzed by Indian aestheticians for centuries. One of the simplest and yet most profound understandings of this process is described by Nandikeshwara in *Abhinaya Darpana,* his treatise on the art of dramatic expression.

> *Where the hand goes, the glance follows.*
> *Where the glance goes, there arises conceptualization.*
> *Where there is conceptualization, there arises emotion.*
> *Out of emotion arises rasa.*

This verse beautifully and succinctly describes the fluid connection between body and spirit, and the transcendent movement that is the essence of Indian classical dance and drama. It begins with the physical dimension of art, its embodiedness, in which the hand represents the entire physical body. The statement that the glance follows the hand might lead one to ask, "Whose glance?" The answer is both the dancer's glance and the glance of the audience. Here her body becomes an act of communication, for, in Indian dance and drama, verbal content is primarily expressed not orally but through a stylized language of gestures. The audience and the dancer are united in the glance, for it is the dancer's task to draw the audience's attention to her gesture and its meaning through the use of her eyes and facial expression.

In the use of this language the dancer's hands represent the sum total of her body language, and also point beyond her body to the realm of the mind, the domain of language and conceptualization. This language in turn gives rise to feeling, for the Hindu worldview recognizes that there can be no thought without feeling. Here *feeling* refers to the associative dimension of experience, the dimension on which all subjectivity is based.

The importance given to subjectivity is a particularly subtle and profound aspect of Indian thought that, until recently, has been intensely resisted in the West. In a sense the main difference between eastern and western philosophies is the western insistence upon the possibility of objective knowledge as the basis of truth. From its earliest formulations eastern thought has insisted on a deeper and more holistic sense of truth, a wisdom that starts from a basic and self-consciousness awareness that all models of reality proceed from the "I," the subjective position. In fact, eastern philosophy has refused to acknowledge anything but a provisional separation between objectivity and subjectivity, the seer and that which is seen. Today, ironically enough, the depth of this basic eastern insight is being borne out by modern science which, having taken objectivity to its most extreme outer and inner limits, is finally recognizing the subjective nature of all human knowledge.

In art there is the possibility of directly experiencing the intimate connection between the inner subjective and outer objective realms, and of overcoming all barriers to their union. This requires conscious reflection upon the workings of the human mind and emotions, a process for which drama provides the most perfect conditions. When this awareness is highly developed there exists the possibility of using that same emotion to move beyond the subjective individual state into a deeper and higher level of consciousness, leading to the ultimate experience of union. Like the state of samadhi, or total absorption, in yoga, the attainment of rasa is a transcendent experience; however, rather than requiring renunciation of one's humanity, drama instead involves a total surrender to one's humanity. Pure rasa is an expansion of the self in which the sum total of all human emotion is encompassed and deeply, profoundly felt. In that moment all particular feelings disappear into the flooding sensation of an all-embracing totality.

Akin to a state of sexual union, the rasa experience involves a total merging into the art, the object of one's contemplation. One moment one is watching the dancer, being drawn ever more deeply in; the next, one is united with her and there is no longer any distinction between the seer and the seen. Without losing any awareness of the self, one is at the same time swept into blissful union.

Anyone who has ever been completely enraptured by art will be able to relate to this process. I myself had one such intense experience of rasa, which at the time took me quite unaware and made me wonder what on earth was happening to me. It was in 1973 in Hyderabad, during my first period of training in the dance. My guru, Natraj Ramakrishna, used to bring troops of Kuchipudi dance artists from the coastal regions of Andhra to the capital in order to help them update their dance dramas for the modern stage. These were performers whose dance was being performed in a folkish style on the dusty roads of the villages, outside the temples. Master, who was researching these older forms of dance, would notate their songs and music and in return would advise them and gift them with new costumes and small amounts of money.

On one such occasion my guru took me along with him. In this dance there were three performers, all male—a father and two sons. The father sang and acted as nattuvangam, reciting the dance syllables and playing the cymbals. One son played the *mrudangam* (drum) while the other son, dressed as a woman, danced and also sang. The drama they performed was the Kuchipudi classic, Bhama Kalapam, the story of Krishna's most beautiful and possessive wife.

Since we were studying this dance in our school, I immediately noticed how different their style was from ours. The costume consisted of a gaudy, well-worn, nine-yard saree and a sash of coarse, heavy bells tied with rope, a crude wig and makeup (tan pancake laid on thick to cover the dark skin of the dancer), exageratedly enlarged eyes, and papier-mâché jewelry.

When the musicians began to sing and the dancer began to move, I was rendered speechless. These villagers were unlike any dancers I had ever seen or heard before. With no microphone their voices filled the huge auditorium. The raw quality of their emotion struck me physically, as if plucking strings along my spinal cord. Breaking out in goosebumps, I slowly felt a heat spread throughout my body. The dance movements bowled me over with their sensuality, an unmediated and unselfconscious eroticism that broke through the limits of the sophisticated urbane Indian culture I had come to accept as normal. I felt my face flush—in what? Embarrassment? Pleasure? Somewhere in the background of this experience my mind feebly reached for categories in which to understand what was happening, while another part of me was just surrendering to it, enjoying the pure sensation of it. At some point I felt my mind totally let go, but it was not a falling back into a kind of unconsciousness. It felt more like an "offering up" of all thoughts to something higher and much more subtle, a felt sense of what the dance was really about: the lover's cry of longing for the beloved, self for highest self, separation for union.

That felt sense blossomed into a fragile lotus, an understanding that I delicately held in my heart as I soared like a kite into the highest reaches of desire. Time stood still as the focus of my concentration narrowed to the point where all that existed in the universe was this dancer, a perfectly transparent symbol of the human soul. As her voice reverberated throughout my body, tears streamed down my cheeks and an orgasmic rush flooded me and held me in rapture until the songs died down. When the performance ended I slowly returned to earth, and to my normal senses.

After the performance I met with the artists in their dressing room. I was shocked to see the contrast between the dancer's stage persona and his ordinary appearance. His name was Suryanarayan, and he was actually an extremely shy person, not much older than I was at the time. Because he and his family were villagers who had never before met a foreigner, they were made extremely self-conscious, but at the same time seemed honored by the attention I paid them, the praise I conveyed through broken Telugu. During our conversation they turned the tables on me, requesting me to perform for them. They wanted me to sing a song from my country, a request that was fairly common in those days. Feeling myself to be a horrible singer, after much persuasion and guilt-tripping on the part of a translator I took a chance on "Those Were the Days," which I delivered with as much confidence as I could muster. They stood and listened, wide-eyed and respectful until the end of the song, which I followed with apologies for what had been a very unequal exchange. From their reactions I could be certain that my little performance did not lead to any transcendent rasa experience for them. Smiling, they graciously commented that our music is "very different" from theirs.

Given what I had gone through during his performance, I could not help but feel some sexual attraction for Suryanarayan, the male dancer who had just laid bare his soul on the stage. This was in spite of the fact that he was rather a plain-looking fellow who, out of costume, could hardly look a woman in the eye. I asked myself to who, exactly, was I feeling attraction? Was I attracted to the male performer behind the female impersonation, or to Satyabhama herself? What was this strange conjunction of raw sexuality and sublime spirituality that scrambles all distinctions of gender and class, high and low culture? And finally, how did Suryanarayan experience his own performance? How I wish I could have climbed inside his body and felt his sensations when, dressed in drag, he enacted the role of Satyabhama.

This became a question I have long since pondered: whether or not the dancer herself can experience rasa even while she is in the midst of displaying emotions (the bhavas). Based on discussions with many dancers, as well as my own experience on the stage, I have arrived at the opinion that the rasa experience is possible even for the performer, but it necessarily takes a different form than that experienced by the audience. For before the artist can achieve unity she must first of all become dualistic.

The artist certainly experiences the particular rasas she portrays; the result is a condition parallel to the state of *dharana,* or total concentration, as described in classical yoga. In this state the dancer's consciousness comes to occupy two positions at once—both that of the artist and that of a witness of her own dance. At some level any dancer has to imaginatively practice this double consciousness in order to conform to an ideal. While keeping track of how a position or movement feels from the inside, she must also imagine how it looks to the audience. In rare cases this can result in an out-of-body experience like the one Natraj Ramakrishna related to me, when he actually saw himself dancing from a viewpoint outside his own body.

Such an experience requires complete involvement in the emotion. According to the way in which we were taught abhinaya by Natraj Ramakrishna, satvika abhinaya, the portrayal of innate expression, requires that the artist actually feel the emotions she portrays. At the same time the artist knows that she is producing the emotion she is feeling. Rasa, or bliss, therefore arises within the dancer when she both displays the feelings, experiencing their essence, and witnesses them as if from outside. At that moment the artist is both the subject and the object, the producer of rasa and the rasika, the enjoyer of aesthetic experience. Indian aesthetics calls for the artist to evolve even further into the ultimate yogic state by transcending this dual consciousness itself. The dancer moves from the individual rasas to "become" pure rasa: there is no longer a differentiation between the producer and the produced, the taster and the taste. Rasa finally evolves into a blissful state of perfect unity.

Once I asked my dance guru, Bala, about the relationship between yoga and dance. She replied, "If someone goes deeply into art, or anything worthwhile that they really enjoy, up to the extent that they forget themselves, they can find the truth through that. In that way dance is a yoga. But in yoga only one person can enjoy the meditation. In dance, if the dancer is fully involved, she can take the entire audience with her to that state of bliss. Yoga means to be fully involved. There is power in it."

The Dream of Myth

Dramatic art therefore functions as a powerful ritual that actually creates that which it describes: a state of transcendence. For this reason the *Natya Sastra* is referred to as the fifth Veda, taking its essential elements from the four main Vedas of the orthodox tradition—songs from the *Sama Veda,* ritual from the *Rig Veda,* abhinaya from the *Yajur Veda,* and rasa from the *Atharva Veda.* However, unlike the other four Vedas that may be read and studied only by the upper castes, the art of drama is accessible to all within the society. Indeed, drama played a central role in both uniting the community and assuring the continuity of tradition. Through the channeling of human emotion into predetermined and prescribed forms, myth and drama were central in defining the religious worldview shared by peasants and kings, merchants and holy men, rich and poor, men, women, and children. On the most basic level, myth and drama functioned as both education and entertainment. But they also had their esoteric dimensions meant only for spiritual initiates, yogis who sought to practically use the images of myth to both alter consciousness and gain access to other worlds.

From the yogic perspective, the subtle, psychic, or emotional body is used to transport oneself to svarga loka, the mythological realm of the gods. This loka, or plane of existence, is understood by yogis as being located within the psychic body, which inhabits (but is not confined to) the physical body. The idea that the gods exist within the human body is a recurrent one within Hinduism; the gods and goddesses of Hindu mythology live in various areas of the body. For example, in Sri Vidya and other tantric systems goddesses are visualized as sitting in specific chakras as protectresses or manifestations of higher energies, each in union with a consort. These goddesses can be understood through mental processes, by reflecting on the symbolic significance of their names and functions within the larger schemata or order. But more important to the tradition is accessing these energies through feeling. By activating subtle emotions through devotional ritual, the devotee taps into these deities' divine realms of bliss and transcendent states of consciousness.

Similarly, many places of pilgrimage frequented by holy men and commoners alike are sites of various episodes from mythology that also find their counterpart within the human body. The Bhagavad Gita, the prebattle scene of the Great War in the Hindu epic Mahabharata, is a prime example. One of the most influential texts of the Hindu tradition, the story describes a struggle for power between two sets of cousins: the five Pandavas, who represent the proverbial good guys, and their out-of-control cousins, the one hundred Kauravas. The story, in which these two sides battle for a kingdom, has many layers of symbolic meaning.

At the beginning of the Bhagavad Gita the two armies are lined up ready to charge at each other when Arjuna, the greatest Pandava warrior, begins to doubt his course of action. Seeing his cousins, brothers, and friends armed to the teeth, most of them destined to die on the battleground, Arjuna turns to his charioteer—who happens to be none other than Krishna, the Supreme Lord himself—and states his refusal to fight. In the next sixteen chapters Krishna gives Arjuna all the reasons why he *must* fight: by doing battle he is upholding dharma, the universal rule of justice. The entire world order depends upon its defense. At the same time Krishna tells Arjuna not to worry for the state of his, or his relative's, eternal souls, for "nothing is created and nothing is destroyed." All are reborn in accordance with their past actions. Arjuna is finally convinced of this when Krishna reveals himself as God in his universal, omnipotent, and omnipresent form, becoming all that is, was, and ever shall be. Having direct experience of the totality of God and eternity, Arjuna is ready to face the limited reality that presents itself to him. He sounds the war cry and the battle begins.

While the story of this battle has come to stand for the larger values of Indian civilization, and the kingdom for the geographic region of the Indian subcontinent, yogis interpret this text entirely as an inner human struggle. The five Pandavas represent the five senses, while the one hundred Kauravas are the objects of the senses. Which will gain control over the self, represented by the supreme warrior Arjuna? It is only when Arjuna has direct experience of God's infinite nature—interpreted by yogis as one's own eternal self, the *atman* or soul, which is one with Brahman, or God—that humankind emerges victorious. According to this interpretation, the Bhagavad Gita illustrates that every moment of every day is a battle for control over the tyranny of the myriad sensory objects, but by defintion it is a battle we cannot avoid.

To give another example, Shiva and Shakti, representing the cosmic male and female principles, are mythological and philosophic concepts common to both yoga and Indian classical dance. Shiva Nataraja, or Dancing Shiva, is not only the patron deity of the dance in India; his dance encompasses the entire creation, whether manifest as internal consciousness or the outer universe.

In Puja, the prayer dance we perform at the beginning of our class, a Sanskrit *sloka* (verse) describes Nataraja's cosmic form:

He whose body is the whole universe,
Whose speech incorporates all utterance, poetry, and
    literature,

*Whose ornaments are the sun and the moon,
To that Shiva I bow.*

In the form of Nataraja, Shiva's dance embodies his own shakti, his active, feminine principle. In other depictions Shiva dances his *tandavam* (masculine) dance alongside his Shakti consort, who dances *lasya,* the complementary graceful feminine form. In yet other iconographic images, the active feminine principle becomes dominant and Shakti, in the form of Kali, the destructress, dances on Shiva's prone and passive body.

Because dance represents sacred action in Hindu mythology, dance imagery is not confined to Shiva and Shakti. Many of the major Hindu gods are depicted as dancing. Ganesh, the elephant-headed god, dances with his big round belly. Krishna, the incarnation of the great Lord Vishnu, Preserver of the Universe, dances on the hood of the snake Kalika to show that he has defeated Kalika in battle. This is a mythological representation of the evolution of culture from earlier stages—represented by the snake—to the pastoral stage. More famous still is Krishna's dance with the *gopis* (milk maidens) in Brindaban, the enchanted forest. With the gopis Krishna performs the Ras Lila, the "Play of Bliss" or "Play of Pure Emotion." In a circle he dances with each woman simultaneously, making each think that he is dancing only with her.

While volumes have been written about the cosmic significance of Krishna's sacred dance, in short the Ras circle dance symbolizes the mandala, the totality of the created universe. The mandala, or sacred circle, is the primary archetypal pattern that reflects the holistic Hindu understanding of the cosmos. The mandala is the most abstract level on which the subtle body itself is brought into the larger picture, so that the yogi's body becomes identified with the entire cosmos. But there are mandalas within mandalas. In tantric yoga systems the chakras located at various points along the spinal column are visualized as energy mandalas while the sahasrara, or "thousand-petaled lotus," represents the crown chakra, the master mandala of the human organism that commands all the other chakras within the body. In Indian dance, even on the most basic or physical level, mandalas are important. They are incorporated into the basic movements, created by the rotating position of the arms, legs, and feet, and the movement of the torso and neck. Taken as a whole, the entire body is itself a mandala.

Each of the major deities of the Hindu pantheon has its own mandala in which it occupies the center. As such, Krishna is the infinitely loving and incredibly beautiful incarnation of the Supreme Lord Vishnu, the embodiment of the principle of sustenance—all that attracts and keeps us attached to earthly existence—while the gopis represent the human soul whose basic state is that of desire or longing for the divine in its manifest form. The gopis experience sringara rasa, romantic love, and its full range of bhavas or variations of feelings in their love for Krishna.

Krishna is the archetypal lover and hero, the immanent personification of transcendent love and desire. With the emphasis placed on bhakti, or devotion, in Krishna worship, medieval Vaishnavism (Vishnu worship) gave rise to a revolution in the arts throughout India. Under its influence not only did the dramatic arts flourish, but religious sadhana based on drama and aesthetics became available to all castes within the society. Many ascetic orders were created that based their meditation techniques on acting out scenes from the life of Krishna or imagining themselves a part of his world.

Similarly, every classical Indian dance tradition came to include a plethora of dances based on the themes of Krishna's life. Odissi dance from Orissa in eastern India is famous for its dances based on the Gita Govinda, the story of the love between Krishna and Radha, his cowherd girlfriend. The devadasis and court dancers throughout South India used to perform *padams* and *javalis* (poetic dance compositions) centering on a heroine's longing for Krishna. The Kuchipudi tradition originated as a type of Bhagavata Mela, a dramatic sadhana in which themes from the life of Krishna were acted out by Brahman males. Many of the most important Kuchipudi dramas were written by Siddhendra Yogi, who is given credit for being the "father" of Kuchipudi dance drama, and whose compositions constitute the style's traditional base. His most famous composition is the Bhama Kalapam, the story of Krishna's possessive wife.

It is not hard to understand why the Bhama Kalapam drama came to be so popular. It depicts the entire gamut of feelings and emotions associated with romantic love: shyness, pride, longing, jealousy, and so on, all emotions immediately accessible to the audience. When performed by men dressed as women, Bhama Kalapam provided an opportunity for men to identify with women's emotions, to exaggerate them, to empathize at some times and to make light of them at others, all within the context of a larger symbolic meaning. For throughout the play Krishna is continually described in terms that emphasize his transcendent or cosmic qualities as well as his earthly ones. Traditionally, the role could be played in an overtly erotic manner without losing its spiritual essence. Today, with the advent of modern standards of decorum, when women perform this role they are expected to be more circumspect, to play the role straight and to enact the necessary emotions without displaying immodesty. Therefore the ideal devotional aspects of Bhama's character are emphasized over her human weaknesses, which makes the drama less colorful than when it was once performed by men.

Witnessing the Drama

Through religious-based drama Indian culture has traditionally honored the emotions as a divine realm where human values originate and play themselves out. It is not that the Hindu gods always provide the best example for human behavior, but the mistakes they make are nonetheless those that humans can learn from. Drama as a whole offers great insight into the human condition. Through drama we develop sensitivity for the human condition and compassion for others. At the same time, drama develops wisdom. No matter how involved we are in the emotions being portrayed on the stage, at least a part of us remains detached knowing that it is all a play that we can leave at any point. When witnessing a stage or screen production, there is freedom in knowing that the pain, horror, fear, or other unpleasant emotions that threaten to overwhelm us are not "real"; at the same time we can choose to identify with those emotions that give us pleasure, insight, or whatever else we are desiring to vicariously experience.

Although Indian dramatic theory clearly differentiates between the rasas (aesthetic experience) and actual human emotions, drama may nonetheless be taken as a metaphor for the psychic body, for the life of the emotions. In India the drama of life is structured by the traditional myths people grow up with, while in the West we are much freer to choose our individual roles. Nonetheless, we have our own cultural myths that program us to play out the drama of our lives in certain predetermined ways. The archetypal themes that structured the myths of our ancient forefathers adapt themselves to the modern context and reappear in our films and television serials and in our family lives and other relationships. From fairy tales to national prime-time news, we see the same stories of human desire playing themselves out in new variations on old themes.

Yet we need not necessarily become enslaved by the patterns of the collective culture. Through conscious awareness of the workings of the drama itself, some reflection on how the drama is produced, we can attain a degree of immunity from overidentifying with any given plot. This can be achieved through what I call "yoga of the emotions," a therapeutic application of dramatic principles in everyday life. Just as we exercise our muscles or physical body, we can exercise our emotions or psychic body through some basic techniques taken from Hindu drama.

The main goal of practicing a yoga of the emotions is to become not only the main performer but also the main audience of your own life's drama. I call this the development of witness consciousness, the ability to observe your own emotions, even in the most intense moments, with a certain amount of dispassion and detachment. In witness consciousness you are fully involved in life, yet at the same time some small part of your consciousness is reserved for reflection on the fact that all of life is a passing drama that has a beginning, a middle, and an end. Of course in those moments when we are ecstatic, blissfully happy, or feeling at peace we will be least likely to want to think that the feelings will pass. It is understandable that during those moments we choose to forget that life is only a drama. This is fine as long as it lasts, but unhappiness or dissatisfaction easily arises when the good times end. It is when pain and misery strike us or those we care about that viewing life as a drama can help restore perspective and psychic equilibrium.

Relative detachment is not the same as being hard-hearted or numb. Emotions are an essential part of being human. The more we try to repress our feelings in order to not feel pain, the more pain they bring when they finally escape our censorship. Traditional yoga teaches that one should always maintain a state of equilibrium. When things go well we should not feel too much joy, nor should we become too disappointed when things go wrong.

The yoga of the emotions that I am advocating here is somewhat more practical than its traditional formulation for those of us who are not ready to distance ourselves from the world. Rather than holding up an ideal of absolute detachment, it takes for granted that we will at times lose ourselves in our feelings, either positive or negative. Through witness consciousness we can quickly regain our balance once again.

The other side of witness consciousness or detachment is the ability to feel and express emotion in healthy and appropriate ways. Disease does not arise from feeling too much emotion, even if the emotions are negative; it arises from swallowing or repressing emotions that cannot be easily digested, and which then cause mental and emotional constipation, upsetting the functioning of the psychic body. Such disturbance manifests as depression or other more severe forms of mental illness that rob us of our full humanity. To be complete human beings we need to experience the full range of human emotions and to keep them in motion.

A good antidote for too many negative emotions is the conscious invocation and practice of positive feelings. I have developed the following exercises based on techniques from Indian dance training, in order to actively and consciously invoke emotions and observe their effect on the psyche. Using these questions we can come to familiarize ourselves with our emotions and to keep them moving. The meditations also help us to gain control over the manner in which we express our emotions to the outside world, hence influencing the feedback we receive from others.

Earlier in this chapter I demonstrate the nine archetypal rasas of Indian aesthetics. Gazing into a mirror, invoke these emotions one by one. You can either internalize what you see in these photographs or simply repeat the names of each of the rasas, making an effort to express that feeling on your face. As you do so, ask yourself the following questions:

- Does the way your face appears reflect the emotion you are invoking? How big is the gap between what you are feeling inside and what you are showing externally?
- Does this emotion come naturally to you? Does it feel uncomfortable? Is this emotion dominant in your life? Do you consciously or unconsciously display this feeling through your face and body language in your daily interactions? Do you want to?
- Reflect on the relationship between emotion and the breath. You will find that in order to invoke a certain emotion you have to change your breathing pattern. As you practice displaying each of the nine rasas, consciously observe the ways in which you are breathing. In yoga, a technique for gaining control over one's emotions is to regulate the breath. Even in the West it is a common practice to take three deep breaths when you are angry or upset. "Witness consciousness" begins with examining our own breathing patterns, not only in meditation but also in the midst of various emotional states.
- What memories or thoughts does this rasa trigger? How deeply does the appearance of a feigned emotion resonate within you? During this part of the exercise, make no attempt to repress any bhavas, or related emotions, that arise in conjunction with a given rasa; instead, let yourself act out whatever comes up while simultaneously witnessing the drama. Just as in meditation, when images arise in the mind one should not try to suppress them but instead practice letting go of them. With practice, this waking meditation will be helpful to you when you find yourself immersed in a life drama. Through witness consciousness you can gain control over the emotions by letting go of them as they arise. Later, if there are still residual effects, instead of acting out with other people you can clear your emotions by expressing them when you are alone. If necessary you can go to a private place and scream, cry, or punch a pillow—this is greatly preferable to dumping negativity on those around you. Such expression can have a powerfully therapeutic effect by inducing a catharsis, a free flow of feeling that cleanses the *manas*, the mind/heart.
- Finally, end your yoga of the emotions session with santa rasa, the feeling of peace. Various commentators on Indian aesthetics have argued that santa rasa is the primary rasa from which all other rasas originate, and into which all other rasas finally merge. Making your face peaceful, let peacefulness permeate your entire body. Keeping your eyes half-open, let santa rasa lead you deeply into witness consciousness.

SIX

The Dance of the Yogini
Tantric Dimensions of Indian Classical Dance

As a form of religious expression, Indian classical dance is highly determined by the cultural values and norms of the larger Hindu tradition. For this reason I believe that if Indian classical dance is to be understood as a kind of yoga, it must be realized that at its core it is a tantric yoga. To explain why this is so, tantra must be examined within the context of the historical development of the Hindu religion.

As with yoga, and dance in any culture, Indian classical dance reflects the central values of the culture in which it developed. These values in turn reflect man-made hierarchies associated with the development of civilizations. As the archaeological remains of Mohenjo Daro and Harappan civilizations indicate, the Indian subcontinent developed agriculture and urban centers involving worldwide trade routes and intercultural contacts at a very remote date. This suggests that from ancient times India was the home of a highly sophisticated urban culture; this was so even before the arrival of the Aryans, those intruders from the northwest whose culture came to dominate the region around the second millennium B.C. Although they undoubtedly borrowed elements from the preexisting culture they supplanted, the Aryans are given credit for establishing the Vedic religion, a highly hierarchical and ritually ordered worldview that remains the more orthodox basis of Sanatan Dharma, or Hinduism, as it is called today.

All cultures use religious means to create patterns out of chaos, to bring that which is yet unknown into a universe of meaning and control. For the earliest Aryan settlers, the main ritual by which the world was literally "created" was the *yajna*, or sacrificial fire. By this ritual various plant and food substances were offered to the gods of nature and the cosmos to the accompaniment of Sanskrit chants, mantras believed to be endowed with magical sound qualities. These Vedic rituals were performed and maintained by a class of hereditary priests called Brahmans. Their name refers to those whose purpose it was to understand and invoke the highest concept of being and ultimate reality, Brahman.

In light of this transcendent principle, the Brahmans conceived of a highly ordered universe in which hierarchy was a central feature: "evolved" culture took precedence over "primitive" nature, "culturally oriented" male took precedence over "natural" female, that which was subtle was regarded to be greater than that which was perceived as purely physical or material. In delineating the universe in this manner these principles were never meant to be understood in simple opposition to each other, for the ideal was always that of an ordered whole in which each part had its role to play relative to its complementary other. With this acute insight into the nature of the universe, Brahmanical Hinduism displayed a spiritual depth unmatched by the world's other religious traditions. But its ideal of holistic interconnectedness was difficult to put into practice, a fact most clearly reflected in the history of the caste system, the social structure that grew out of the Vedic concept of *varna*.

Varna refers to the classification of human beings based on the Vedic myth of Purusha, the first man who sacrificed himself in order to create the cosmos. According to the myth, from Purusha's head sprang Brahmans, the priestly class; from his shoulders came the Kshatriyas, or warriors; from his thighs were born the Vaishyas, or merchants; and from his feet came the Sudras, or laborers. It is important to note that outcastes, those tribal inhabitants of the subcontinent who predated the Aryan presence, do not even figure within this cosmic order. Not even accorded a fully human status, they are relegated to the realm of chaos.

Because Brahmans themselves represented the pole of transcendence within the social hierarchy, they saw it as their ritual duty to keep the hierarchical order intact by exerting ideological control over those below them in the Purusha cosmology. But they could not have maintained their position without the cooperation of the other two "twice-born" or upper castes, the Kshatriyas and the Vaishyas. Although numerically in the minority, all three upper castes cooperated to maintain dominance over the low-caste Sudra laborers. The Kshatriya rulers, kings drawn from the second-highest varna, depended on the Brahmans' priestly powers to maintain the order of their kingdom, while the Vaishya merchants depended upon both the rulers and the priests. Therefore, under the protection of the warrior-kings and with the patronage of merchants, over thousands of years the Brahmans increasingly systematized, codified, and refined their vision of society and the cosmos, a worldview within which they continually maintained their own privileged status.

Undoubtedly the maintenance of a class of men dedicated to intellectual and spiritual pursuits resulted in rich cultural dividends: India today boasts the world's most ancient and highly developed continuous literate culture. Long before the European enlightenment gave birth to modern science, Vedic Hinduism engaged in its own version of scientific conceptualization and gave birth to mathematics, astronomy, alchemy, and medicine, as well as to such inner-oriented disciplines as philosophy, yoga, and the visual and performing arts of sculpture, painting, dance, music, and drama.

However, this intellectual development came with a price: it opened a gap between nature and spirit and between male and female, one that has led to the denigration of both nature and the feminine in the name of "higher" truths. Such disparity is characteristic of all great civilizations, and we can see ample evidence of this phenomenon throughout the world today. In mainstream Indian culture we see it in the low status afforded women and tribals, as well as a general disregard for the environment. So it is that when we reflect upon the history of Hinduism, we necessarily find ourselves questioning some of its most central values.

As a culture, India has prided itself on its spirituality. As is the case with all major world religions, that which lies at the heart of spirituality is the notion of transcendence, envisioned spatially as a movement out of one level of being into a higher state. Historically and philosophically, transcendence may be conceptualized as a process of increasing consciousness, the development of self-conscious reflection, the notion that there exists a spirit or force that impels human beings away from, above and beyond, one's given condition: that condition being "nature," the state into which one is born unaware. In this formulation, nature, often equated with raw matter or materiality, is that which conscious spirit defines itself in opposition to. Therefore spirit and matter, or spirit and nature, become increasingly polarized, opening a gaping hole in the whole.

As it is in many highly developed cultures, and in India as well, this polarization of nature and spirit manifests itself profoundly in the relationship between male and female. Within the earliest Vedic worldview it is notable that all major deities are male, while the few references to feminine deities in the Vedas refer to less differentiated forces of nature. Thus, from the beginning male and high caste were equated with transcendence and order, while female and low caste were associated with nature and chaos, that which needed to be controlled. This is most apparent within mainstream (popular) polytheistic Hinduism, where goddesses may be classified under two broad categories: those who have husbands, hence their power is under the control of the larger male social order, and those who are independent and hence pose a potential danger to society and the cosmos.

Lakshmi, the goddess of wealth, fertility, and general auspiciousness, is always married to Vishnu, the Lord of Preservation, the model of the Divine King, the supreme ruler who upholds the social order. With few exceptions, in myths and iconographic depictions Lakshmi's character is always portrayed as that of the ideal wife sitting at her husband's side, or even massaging his feet as he reclines on his serpent bed. Because she knows her place, their status as a couple is always harmonious, the very picture of marital bliss. However, the Great Goddess Parvati, the consort of Lord Shiva, Lord of the Beasts, Master Yogi, and Cosmic Dancer, displays more ambiguous characteristics. To become Shiva's consort in the first place, Parvati has to distract him from his meditation in the Himalayas. After their marriage they engage in sessions of lovemaking on Mount Kailash that last for aeons, but the myths also portray them in various kinds of discussions, competitions, and disagreements, many of them both humorous and profound.

In a series of incarnations Parvati takes the form of myriad goddesses, some of them unmarried and independent. For example, as Durga, the warrior-goddess, she defeats various male demons, including Mahisasura, the Buffalo Demon, who lusts after her. Durga is the form of the goddess worshiped by kings, who invoke her fierce energy in battle. But there is danger in calling up her power as portrayed in her most radical incarnation, that of Kali, the Timeless Destroyer, goddess of death. A common myth relates how Kali, on a rampage, becomes so involved in her dance of destruction that she does not know how to stop. Soon the gods are fearful that the entire world will be turned into a cremation ground. Only Shiva can stop her, so he lays down on the ground to bear the brunt of her wrath. When she accidentally steps on him, Kali immediately realizes what she has done and bites her outstretched tongue in shame. This myth, which seeks to explain Kali's lolling tongue, demonstrates the Hindu belief that the destructive aspect of female energy must be kept within limits by male principles of control.

Like Durga, Kali is an unmarried virgin, but she is nonetheless connected to Shiva, the Lord of Destruction, representing his most wrathful shakti, or manifest power. In the temples of both Durga and Kali, the goddess stands at the center of the sanctum while her consort, Shiva, is most often housed separately in a nearby shrine in the iconic image of a *lingam,* a male phallus.

These forms of the goddess speak to divisions within the society and attitudes toward the feminine even today. Lakshmi is worshiped primarily by upper-caste devotees, while the most terrifying forms of the goddess are most popular among the low castes: anthropological and archaeological evidence suggests that the terrifying goddesses of Hinduism, as well as the phallus worship associated with Shiva, are drawn from the orgiastic tribal and Dravidian cultures that predated and greatly influenced Vedic religion. The distinctions between forms of the goddess based on social location demonstrate that in Hinduism, as in many traditional societies, the fear that sexuality will disturb the social order becomes the justification for control of feminine power. The higher the caste the more control is exerted, as upper-caste women are by breeding and socialization expected to conform to greater restrictions.

Nonetheless, because of their ability to give birth, all women, regardless of caste, become associated in Hinduism with raw nature, materiality, and sexuality, and are therefore ideally kept under control. The male social order exerts its power most importantly over women's wombs—their sexuality and reproductive powers are controlled through arranged marriages within caste bounds and strict separation of the genders. It is not that Brahmanical Hinduism denies women's power or sexuality. It actually worships women's sexual power as the goddess herself, calling her Shakti, the power of creation. But at the same time the tradition seeks to keep Shakti under male control, and to harness that energy toward socially reproductive goals. As a result, at the same time that motherhood and the feminine qualities of servitude and selflessness are paid lip service in the name of the goddess, the social reality is that living women are feared and denigrated, and often become victims of degradation, abuse, and worse.

The polarization of nature and spirit shows itself even within the most sophisticated philosophical formulations that flourished within the Brahmanical tradition. In the more orthodox formulations, which counsel renunciation or asceticism as the highest path to spiritual liberation (moksha, or release from the divided state of manifestation), the feminine has been cast simply in the role of *prakriti,* "nature," "matter," that which needs to be renounced or transcended in order to reach the highest goal of moksha. However, Hinduism encompasses much more than its Vedic, orthodox formulation. Despite its claim to eternal and unchanging truth, the Brahmanical worldview did not go unchallenged. The resurgence and reformulation of pre-Aryan elements, the rise of devotionally centered bhakti cults, and other reactions against the highly ritualistic Brahmanical order played an essential and creative role in revitalizing Indian culture and fed into the mix that Hinduism is today. In a dynamic dance of myth and history characterized by invasions and intercultural contact, new elements were constantly introduced, while others that had been temporarily submerged resurfaced and were incorporated into the larger order, leading to important changes and developments. Hence, despite the highly normative principles set down in Brahmanical texts, Indian culture has always been a living reality constantly adapting itself to a changing world.

Tantra and the Goddess Within

From within the framework of Vedic orthodoxy we can begin to understand the role that tantrism played in Indian culture, for the tantric traditions have been the major catalyzing force in a struggle for alternative values within Hinduism. From thousands of Sanskrit texts called the Tantras we come to know about this pervasive religious movement, which began in the early centuries A.D., peaked around the tenth century, and went underground during the period of Muslim rule, yet which continues even today as an undercurrent within Hinduism. Surviving tantric texts show that at the time tantrism flourished there existed thousands of independent cults (here defined as a community of initiates associated with a lineage of teachers or gurus) centered on the ritual invocation of a particular deity, male or female, or sometimes both in union. The forms of these deities varied, but each was invoked as a reflection of not only the cosmos but the highest self. The tantric worldview seeks to bridge the gap opened by the polarization of spirit and matter, and uses various techniques to do so. Through the use of sacred sound and sacred geometric diagrams, such as mandalas, the guru initiated the tantric adept into rituals, visualizations, and deepening states of meditation in order to reveal the limitless nature of consciousness. While techniques and formulations varied, all tantric lineages shared a common goal: the quest for ultimate realization, the nondual knowing of inner self and outer universe as one.

It is important to realize that the tantric lineages have never stood in open and direct opposition to the orthodox Vedic worldview; nonetheless, they have presented a challenge to many dominant Brahmanical values. This may be due to the fact that tantra represents the resurgence and reinterpretation of older, pre-Aryan religious elements that assert themselves within the framework of Vedic Hinduism. These elements, which have survived most predominantly in South Indian Dravidian culture, and in different forms in the remaining tribal communities of the subcontinent, involve the worship of snakes, terrifying forms of the Mother Goddess, and the phallus; spirit possession; human sacrifice; and other orgiastic rites. These shamanic and fertility-based practices represent the oldest substratum of religion in both India and the world as a whole, and are transformed and reinterpreted as they reemerge within the context of Brahmanical Hinduism, taking on symbolic meanings that challenge the Brahmanical worldview even as they revitalize it.

Specifically, through tantra's conscious invocation of the feminine principle, its celebration of the powers of nature and sexuality, and its refusal to limit its community of initiates to Brahmans or even to upper castes, tantra provides an alternative to the values of Brahmanical orthodoxy. Undoubtedly tantra shares the same goal as Vedic Hinduism—a spiritual liberation conceived of as release from limited awareness into Supreme Consciousness—but tantrism questions the orthodox conception of how to achieve that goal. In fact, it denies any clear dichotomy between means and goal, between the immanent, created world and transcendent, "spiritual" reality. Those forces that are regarded within the orthodox formulation as most binding—the source of our deepest attachments: nature, creation, sexuality, the feminine—become the most potent means of liberation within the tantric worldview. Instead of renouncing the world in order to achieve a state of consciousness beyond, tantra embraces the totality of creation as a reflection of the highest self, denying duality in its quest for ultimate unity. Tantra attempts to restore to Hinduism the wholeness that has been lost in the polarization of spirit and nature.

Certainly tantra is the underground current that has sustained the feminine principle within the larger Hindu world. While specific tantric traditions have largely remained esoteric cults, secret sources of power meant only for initiated adherents, tantric elements are nonetheless present throughout the culture, appearing most markedly in popular forms of shaktism (goddess worship). In tantra-inspired shaktism, the feminine principle is the primary means by which liberation is attained. *Shaktas* worship the goddess as Mother, celebrating woman's life-giving powers, but they do not limit her to that role. They recognize the full range of woman's qualities, her connecting nature that weaves life with death, fertility with pleasure, experience with wisdom. The goddess is simultaneously the Supreme Mother, Lover, and Goddess of Time and Death. As nature she liberates man out of narrow, limited existence, from the realm of opposites into the realm of nondual, transcendent union. As the highest creative principle her image teaches us that light and dark, male and female, good and evil, are not opposites but complementary. The darkness of the womb, whether in birth or death, is the source of the light of awareness.

The Goddess as Womb

For transcendence to take place there must be fertility: If there is no creation, there is nothing to transcend. For this reason, fertility takes on many layers of meaning in Hinduism. It does not refer only to sexual reproduction; it stands for creation, and creativity on all levels. In India the most common representation of this larger sense of fertility is the *kalasa,* or sacred water pot, a ritual object that traces its roots to the ancient past.

For thousands of years and throughout the country, a kalasa made of brass or clay, topped with mango leaves and a coconut and decorated with yellow turmeric and red *sindur,* has been used to represent the goddess as watery womb. This is the primary representation of the goddess used in Devi puja (goddess-worship) ceremonies. The association between the goddess and water likely dates to prehistory: The equation of the water pot with a primordial Earth Goddess is obvious, since from time immemorial the development of entire civilizations rested on the lowly water pot. Not only is the water pot symbolic of the womb of life, but without containers for water human beings would be unable to move any distance from rivers or lakes. In archaeological excavations the migrations of various groups are traced primarily through the shards of pottery vessels they left behind. Throughout the ancient world these pots are often found buried at prehistoric megolithic sites and in the ruins of temples, many of which were located at the crossroads of the earliest human footpaths. It is therefore no wonder that the sacredness of rivers and water is such a well-established aspect of religious life in India, dating from the Mohenjo Daro and Harappan cultures. Just as the lingam represents the aniconic form of Shiva, the male principle, so does the water vessel represent the goddess as womb in abstract form.

As a symbol, the womb does not represent just the power of creation or immanence; it more accurately stands for immanence *and* transcendence, and their ultimate inseparability. In the *agamic* tradition (texts that prescribe the art and science of temple building) the innermost chamber or sanctum sanctorum of a temple, the place where the main deity is housed, is called the *garbha griha,* or "womb abode." One of the twelve Sanskrit names for the sun is *hiranya garbha,* or the "golden womb" (the source of all life being associated with the color golden yellow, while the moon is associated with soma [a ritual drink], the color white, and male semen). The term *hatha,* as in hatha yoga, is the conjoining of *ha,* the feminine energy of the sun, and *tha,* the male energy of the moon. In this case it is the feminine energy that is the primary and self-generating creative power, while the moon represents reflective consciousness.

The kalasa, or water pot, is a supremely tantric symbol. In tantric ritual involving actual or symbolic sexual intercourse, the female is known as the *patra,* or "container" that holds the life-giving waters, while the male is associated with the seed, or that which is contained. For creation to take place male and female sexual fluids have to mix, and they must also be given a space, a container, in which to flourish—a literal ground of being. In the tantric worldview, woman's body, the physical ground of being for the origin of human life, is symbolically equated with the earth, the ground of humanity's being. But on a deeper level, woman is the manifestation of the goddess herself, the totality of creation. The goddess as womb not only symbolizes the ground of being of earthly creation but on the cosmic level encompasses the entirety of universal creation; hence, she is consciousness itself. Both transcendent and immanent, the goddess as womb represents the continual re-creation of the universe through conscious awareness—the union of opposites—symbolized, enacted, and realized through the tantric ritual act of sexual union.

Tantric Dimensions of Indian Dance: Eroticism and the Sacred Womb

Like an underground spring, the tantric traditions have in a sense "grounded" the transcendent spirituality of Brahmanical Hinduism, and are probably the main reason why sexuality has retained a dimension of sacredness within the culture. Temple complexes throughout India are covered with erotic sculpture, Konarak and Khajuraho being the most famous examples. Here, alongside sensuous dancers and musicians, one finds amorous couples, triples, and entire groups, both animal and human, depicted in uninhibited sexual play. In the modern era these representations present something of a puzzle to most Hindus, and various theories have been used to try to explain their significance. But one thing is perfectly clear from the lyricism of these forms, from the graceful smiles that play on the lips of these entwined lovers even after centuries of being ravished by rain, wind, and

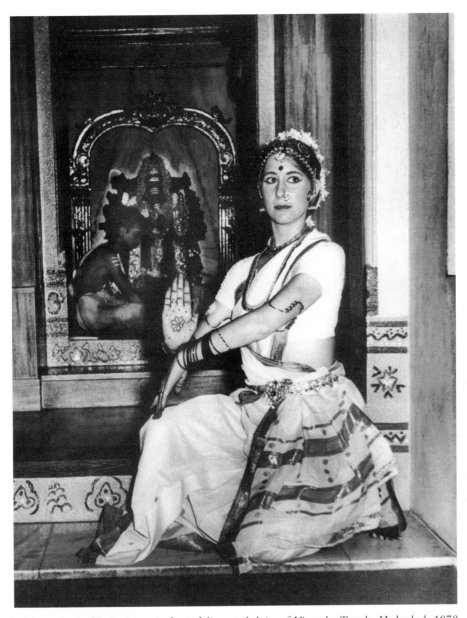

Striking a classic "blessing" pose in front of the central shrine of Vinayaka Temple, Hyderabad, 1978. The traditional temple dancer played an important role by dancing in front of the deity at several points in the daily ritual cycle. A symbol of fertility and good fortune, she held a respected place in the life of the temple. Photograph by G. Krishna.

sun: There is absolutely no sense of shame associated with this sexuality.

Perhaps to fully understand the purpose of these erotic portrayals one must imagine the subjective experience of the pilgrims who once traveled tremendous distances to worship at these great temples. The sheer quantity of these images, arranged in multiple layers on the outer walls of the temples, gives the appearance that the walls themselves are teeming with life. All this activity contrasts greatly with the stark simplicity and quiet of the temple's interior. As the devotee moves from the outside of the temple to the inner womb chamber, all the decorative trappings, representing the world of the senses, finally fall away to reveal the supremely transcendent beauty of the deity that sits majestically at the center of the temple.

This movement from outer to inner world, from creation to transcendence, equates sensual sexuality with the outer realm of creation. At the center that union finds its moment of complete balance, transforming itself into a divine and mystical joining of eternal male and female. To see these two realms as divorced from one another would be to miss the point entirely, for the inner and outer worlds are two poles of the same continuous, nondual reality, each drawing its identity from its complementary opposite. The temple is a cosmos in and of itself and represents the totality of all that is. The stillness at the center extends outward and infuses the activity taking place on the outer walls with its sacredness.

At the great temple complexes of India, the sites of both Vedic and tantric rituals, pilgrims came to pray both for the fulfillment of worldly desires and for spiritual liberation. It was here that they came to have the darshan (sacred vision) of not only the god in the temple but the goddess as well. And it was here that they found her not only sculpted in stone but also living in the form of the temple dancer. It is no coincidence that, on the temple walls, the solitary dancer takes her place amidst lovemaking couples, and that within the temple the living devadasi danced in front of the image of the god, offering her dance in order to bring fertility to the land.

Devadasis danced in the innermost sanctum of the temple in front of the deity, waving a brass *kalasa,* a water pot with a burning oil wick on top. Sexuality, represented by the burning flame, sits atop the watery vessel, representative of the womb of life. This sacred pot lamp, as well as the devadasis themselves, represented the Great Goddess in her many aspects, most explicitly Lakshmi. For Lakshmi was the goddess of not only human fertility but the fertility and prosperity of the land, particularly the geographic area or kingdom in which the temple functioned as a ritual and cultural center. This concept of the productivity and wealth of the land extended into a more general and intangible cultural notion of "auspiciousness," "luckiness," or "fruitfulness." The notion of auspiciousness is still a central part of Hindu religion and art. In the modern era the Indian classical dancer in many ways replaces the devadasi as a symbol of this concept, which is why, in a modern secular context, Indian dance programs are often arranged to be held at weddings, inaugural functions, and other kinds of public ceremonies. Even today the dance continues to invoke blessing energy on any event of importance.

The Dancer as Yogini

While it is a well-established and historical fact that devadasis were regarded as living symbols of the goddess's shakti, or life-giving power, the question arises as to whether or not temple dancers were also living yoginis, women whose primary function within tantrism was to represent the goddess in her ultimate transcendent function—as the embodiment of wisdom and liberation. Although scant historical evidence of this aspect of tantrism survives into the modern age, tantric texts and archaeological evidence both attest to the role of

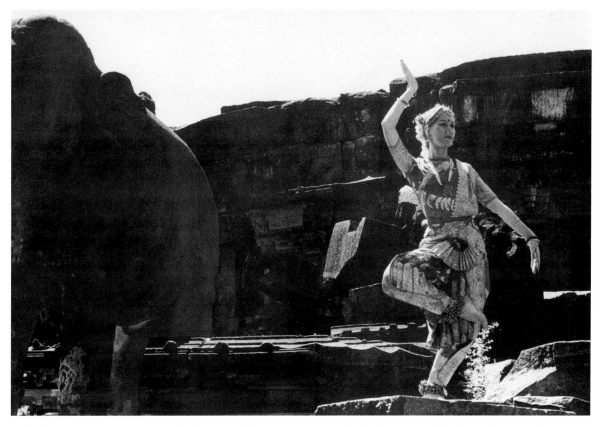

Dancing among the ruins. The Indian dancer is heir to a long lineage of female religious specialists. Just as the devadasi came to replace the yogini as the embodiment of feminine spiritual power, today's classical dancer continues to play a powerful symbolic role in Hindu religious life. Photograph taken in 1978 at Ramappa temple in Palempet, Andhra Pradesh, a major center for dance during the tenth century. Photograph by Shyam.

yoginis in tantric cults. Like the siddhas or male tantric adepts, heroic humans who attained such extraordinary powers through both Hindu and Buddhist tantric practices that they became legends in their own lifetimes and were attributed with the powers of living gods, so too do the tantric texts tell of yoginis, female embodiments of wisdom who inhabited particular geographical locales and who also were believed to have extraordinary powers.

Like the siddhas, yoginis too have developed into the form of lower-level goddesses, usually sixty-four in number, and are portrayed as sculpted images in the few surviving yogini temples. The architecture of yogini temples is distinctive—a mandala-shaped circular form, open to the sky but perhaps once covered with thatch. This shape is suggestive of *panchamakara* tantric rituals in which couples sat in a circle and offered the "five Ms" to their guru ancestral lineage: *mamsa* (meat), *matsya* (fish), *mudra* (parched grain), *madya* (wine), and *maithuna* (sexual intercourse). The architecture may also harken back to earlier thatched tribal structures, which are round in shape. The tribal origins of these sexual rituals can only be guessed at, but there is no question that many of the

THE DANCE OF THE YOGINI ❦ 171

goddesses of early tantra are borrowed directly from tribal regions and have similarly untamed characteristics. Therefore the yoginis present an enigma, even within tantric studies. Some texts describe the yoginis as powerful witches with magical capabilities, while others attribute to them the qualities of deities. Still other texts refer to them as the realized sexual initiatresses of siddhas within specific tantric lineages. One thing we do know is that the yoginis were spiritually powerful and their power was related to their sexuality.

If there are such yoginis living in India today, they are well hidden. They would have to keep their identities secret. In fact, because the term *yogini* has many somewhat dangerous connotations, in Indian culture today a woman ascetic who practices yoga is called Mother—"Amma" or "Mataji"—titles meant to establish their status as a living mother goddess. In this title the maternal aspects are stressed and the sexual dimensions are downplayed or entirely ignored. This has to do with Indian attitudes toward female sexuality, which immediately consider any unmarried or independent woman as sexually suspect.

While no theory linking devadasis and yoginis can be historically proven, given the evidence I believe it is possible that the devadasi came to replace the yogini both as a living female ritual specialist and as a symbol of the goddess and feminine spiritual power. In a sense, just as the fierce yoginis represented a survival of the untamed sexuality of a pre-Aryan tribal goddess who becomes transfigured into an initiator of the heroic tantric siddha, the devadasi represents a more tamed or domesticated version of the same goddess energy. Her Lakshmi, life-giving "culture," is emphasized over her Kali, transcendently erotic "nature." Both are living goddesses, but the goddess has evolved into a benevolent protector of the kingdom—essentially a human creation.

When the wilder, more ecstatic forms of tantra were driven out of India into Nepal and northeastern India, where their traces still exist today, some of their secret practices were hidden in the heart of orthodox Hinduism, and a milder version of tantric symbolism became incorporated into popular temple culture. At the same period of time, "evolving" society no longer had a place for powerful and independent female ascetics like the yoginis. They too were either driven out of the settled areas into the wilderness of the tribal areas (which is why today it is only in Nepal, Assam, and Bengal that you will find traces of these yoginis) or forced into the domestication of the temple complexes.

Yet in the secret tantric traditions that have survived the "evolution" of history within mainstream Hinduism, there is no question that there were devadasis who played the role of sexual partner to tantric practitioners (usually Brahman priests), even if they lost the yogini's original independence. For those who have understood the tantric teachings, I believe that the secret of feminine power has not been entirely lost. Even today, when the devadasi has been expelled from the temple to find her reincarnation on the modern stage, her image still brings together the sacredness of the earth and cosmic transcendence. Embodying both Vedic and tantric attitudes toward the feminine and creation, her dance is still intimately bound to both the deepest and the highest significance of sexuality. Within the image of the devadasi, within the dance of the classical dancer, dances a secret yogini.

SEVEN

Yoga of the Elements
Nature, Culture, and Spirituality

According to Hindu mythology, untamed nature or wilderness is an enchanted realm filled with many categories of wondrous beings, both benign and terrifying. *Yakshis* and *yakshas,* male and female forest spirits worshiped and feared by tribal peoples, were transformed into deities in the Hindu pantheon, and appear in their most powerful forms in the tantric traditions. Likewise, the worship of *nagas* and *naginis,* male and female serpent beings, is among the most ancient of all indigenous practices and figures largely in folk Hinduism and Buddhism. Kundalini is a further (tantric) development of the serpent image representing evolving human consciousness, an unfolding process of transcendence rising out of the earth. Feminine in nature, the tantric Kundalini is an anthropomorphic, psycho-physiological concept: Spirit now resides not only in the external cosmos but within the human body as an energy that rises from the lowest, earth, chakra upward through the higher centers, finally uniting with the crown chakra, the sahasrara or thousand-petaled lotus, at the top of the skull. The skull itself is a powerful image in tantra representing the realm of transcendence, an opening into the inner sky, the infinity of inner space.

The outer sky was also understood to be inhabited by wondrous beings. In the Vedas and the epics, later myths based on Vedic themes, the *apsaras,* or female flying spirits, and *gandharvas,* their male counterparts, were seen riding on the winds and dancing on the waves in rivers and the ocean. Sakuntala, the mother of King Bharata (with whom India shares its indigenous name, Bharata), was the daughter of the apsara Menaka, who became pregnant after seducing the powerful yogi Viswamitra. This story illuminates the fact that, from their earliest beginnings as a civilization, Indians have understood themselves as having been born from a race of powerful and holy "supermen" whose intercourse with nature gave birth to a mighty kingdom. This interpretation is reflected in Indian culture throughout its development in the interplay of Vedic and tantric religious elements. Generally speaking, tantra represents and reinterprets the older religious substratum based on fertility rites, the invocation of the feminine, and a less controlled experience of nature, while Vedic ritual represents cultural evolution, the transcendent conceptualization and ritual manipulation of those same elements under the control of a patriarchal elite.

Nonetheless the common basis of these two streams is nature. Perhaps it is true of all cultures that nature is the starting point that is later taken for granted. Like a mother, nature is our origin, it is what we are literally made of, and yet the very existence of a "father" spirit or transcendent energy renders nature as that which we are transcending, that from which we are continually moving away and over which we must always extend control. From one point of view it seems that culture subsumes nature, taming and transforming it, shaping its patterns into man-made forms. From the orthodox Hindu perspective this ordering of culture is man's most sacred activity, and it is to be achieved by ritual means. The Vedas, sacred verses that describe the nature of the world and man's place in it, also prescribe how these rituals are to be performed. Furthermore, these texts are not open to question because they are considered to be revealed, to have been transmitted from a divine source to the *rishis*, the sages of ancient times.

In an earlier chapter I discussed how this highly developed culture of Brahmanical Hinduism, no less effectively than similar civilizations in the West, opened a chasm between spirit and nature.

Today, just as in the West, India rushes to fill that gap with meaningless objects, mimicking the consumerism that is the hallmark of western development. It is of course not surprising that, like the rest of the world, India would embrace science and technology in its search for progress. The simplistic 1960s cliche that "the East is spiritual, the West is materialistic" fell by the wayside long ago, and was blown to bits with the detonation of India's nuclear bomb. But Indians, and all of us on the planet, *together* must consider just how much we are willing to sacrifice to the new god in whose honor such defensive measures become necessary. I am speaking, of course, about the international market economy, the prime mover of today's brave new world order.

In our postmodern world the market lays siege to the values of the European Enlightenment and traditional cultures alike. For even though, on a crassly material level, science has tortured nature into revealing her secrets, for every technological "advancement" nature reasserts her supremacy in an equally forceful backlash of human and environmental misery. As old hierarchies crumble and the market promises (but does not universally deliver) unlimited material growth and prosperity, human consciousness is undergoing an upheaval unparalleled in history. While those in the East and in other developing countries scramble for the goods promised by modernity, in the West there is a general malaise and emptiness among even the most educated and affluent, and indications of a general disenchantment with both religion and science. At the same time there is a burgeoning of interest in matters of the spirit.

People in the West are increasingly drawing distinctions between religion and spirituality. It is a sign of these tumultuous times that a rash of new religious movements is appearing, even as many traditional religious sects are dying out. For religion largely replicates the traditions of the past while spirituality speaks to the new, marking the presence of the eternal in the here and now. While religion defines itself through doctrine and seeks permanency through institutionalization, spirituality draws from the bottomless wellspring of human creativity, the aesthetic realm of art and mysticism. While religion deals in the "truths" of history, spirituality speaks the language of myth and symbol and recognizes the metaphoric in, and hence the relative quality of, all human conceptualizing: Not only beauty but all else too exists primarily in the eye of the beholder.

Cultural relativism, a humanist perspective that arose within modern social science disciplines, informs today's awareness that there is no one truth, but instead there are many truths that need to somehow coexist if a variety of peoples and cultures are to live peaceably on the planet. The bane of religious fundamentalists, cultural relativism may represent much more than a reaction against repressive traditions. Given current world conditions, cultural relativism marks the beginning of a live-and-let-live approach that may represent a survival instinct on the part of the human species, a psychic adaptive strategy for the contemporary global scenario. While some religions may find it hard to reconcile their exoteric doctrines (particularly their moral codes) with relativity, an expanded notion of spirituality may be capable of bridging the gap between humanism and religion. For spirit is present in the esoteric teachings that lie at the core of all religious traditions. Focusing on individual experience, yet recognizing the limitations inherent in language, spirituality celebrates the metaphor at the heart of finite human experience, and that which manifests in the one shared and most basic impulse common to all religions: a desire for the Absolute, a never-ending reaching for the boundless, an archetypal longing for knowledge of the unknown and yet-to-be discovered—in other words, transcendence of every limiting condition.

Despite cultural relativism there is also a felt need for some kind of common ground, some shared worldview or perspective that translates across cultures, bridging differences of caste, creed, ethnicity, and gender in order to enhance our chances of collective survival. But where can we find this shared vision? Many people believe that we must find it here and now, on our literal common ground, the earth itself. The earth, nature, becomes a powerful spiritual category precisely because at this point, when no single existing religion can speak to the entire world, it is the one thing we all have in common. Furthermore, its future is imperiled. It is no coincidence that the rise of earth-centered spirituality, as well as its symbolic counterpart in Mother Goddess worship, comes at a time when the planet is fast approaching ecological disaster and when our own technology threatens our very continuation as a species. For the first time in human history, thanks to nuclear proliferation, we are now capable of destroying the very terra firma on which we stand. Because we can no longer take her stability, or even her survival, for granted, many look to Mother Earth and those cultures that we perceive as being closer to the earth for the answers to our common dilemma.

Around the world, environmental organizations with secular and political activist agendas address these issues from a variety of perspectives. Often opposed to the very notion of transcendence, many approach the earth and nature from a rational perspective, attempting to ground their ethics on a scientific understanding of biological processes. Some groups are working within the political system, while others practice eco-terrorism in order to defend the planet against rampant development. Despite many environmentalists' rejections of religion, there are nonetheless discernible religious elements present in many of these environmentalist ideologies, the difference being that they substitute the concept of Gaia—the earth, immanent nature—for yesterday's transcendent God or gods. Some believe that in doing so they are returning to an earlier, primordial understanding of what it means to be human.

But there is a danger in this position, which is as unbalanced as the privileging of spirit over nature. Just as radical feminism emerged as a reaction against the hierarchies that have enslaved nature and the feminine, a new order is envisioned that simply reverses the traditional one. To hold all men (or all white men for that matter) responsible for the destruction of the planet is to create a new fascist ideology. Similarly, to deny transcendence or spirit is to reduce the earth to soulless matter, and social reality to what philosopher Ken Wilbur refers to as "the Flatlands," an existential wasteland in which the lowest common denominator holds reign. Even from the point of view of science, as soon as life and its processes are taken into consideration you are again dealing with spirit, hierarchy, and some notion of "evolution" or transcendence. Rather than embrace a set of oppositions that simply reverses the old, a re-visioning of the interrelationship between nature and spirit, between male and female, is called for. It is possible to be both an environmentalist and a feminist without calling for the destruction of all hierarchies, or all traditional structures for that matter.

From the viewpoint of Indian spirituality, that is, within the hitherto esoteric traditions that offer an alternative understanding of the human's place on the planet, there can be no real opposition between immanence and transcendence. From a tantric viewpoint, which takes the higher self as the ultimate reference point and the harmonious interaction of male and female as a central metaphor, culture cannot be understood as separate from nature. Neither can human consciousness be understood as separate from the body, which is after all made up of the same elements as the earth. Male is contained in female and female in male. The very patterns that constitute culture arise from within human consciousness, which is also a part of nature. Instead, culture may be conceived as a projection of universal consciousness, Nature revealing itself to its Self, the self becoming self-aware.

This expanding, evolving nature is the only truly unlimited frontier, and it both exists within the human and is the context within which the human is defined. This nature will never be fully understood by science, controlled by technology, or exhausted through thought or language. Yet it is within the human capacity to experience. Yoga is one of the means by which this becomes possible, by which this *human* nature is revealed. From the viewpoint of religion, yoga is sometimes described as a science, as if this grants yoga some kind of superior legitimacy. But from the viewpoint of spirituality yoga is an art, for yoga is much more than physics which, despite its most mind-blowing theoretical formulations, is nonetheless limited by its concern with objective verification. Yoga is rather "psychics," concerned with subjective human experience whether or not that can be controlled, measured, or replicated, proven, disproven, or marketed for profit. It is an affirmation of the primacy of the eternal now over that which has come before or even that which is yet to come, for our notions of past and future are as limited as any other concepts.

While, undeniably, the goal of yoga is transcendence, that goal can be realized only in the subjective and immanent here and now, and one of the ways that can happen is through a synchronization and harmonization of the human with nature. It is this kind of nature mysticism that is implicit within the tantric traditions.

The Yogini's Nature

In tantra, the body mirrors the cosmos. This is a central premise of yoga, and is also reflected in Indian dance. The correspondence between nature and the cosmos is deified in the image of Lord Nataraja, who hails from nature, the untamed wilderness, as Pasupati, Lord of the Beasts, emerging within culture (orthodox Hinduism) as Shiva, the Master Yogi whose cosmic dance of matter and energy gives form to the entire universe. From the esoteric world of tantra emerges an equally powerful, feminine image of self-awareness: the yogini. Also depicted as dancing, she embodies the entrancing qualities of feminine nature spirits such as yakshinis, naginis, and apsaras, but at the same time manifests the shakti, the power of the Great Goddess. A less distant figure than Nataraja, her dance represents the perfect balance between transcendence and immanence. An image that humans can aspire to, a state of being attainable to both men and women, the yogini is none other than Supreme Wisdom and Conscious Awareness, consort to the gods, guru to humankind.

As an energy, the yogini is not unique to India. From the beginning of time wise men throughout the world found her in the natural world—in forests, in springs, in mountains, and in caves. They knew her as the anima, or soul, reflected as the spirit of the flowing waters, flowering trees, and medicinal plants. In their communion with her she revealed alchemical secrets to the wise men that in the West eventually gave rise to objective science, and in the East, the science of self-knowledge. She taught the world about the transformation of both matter and the psyche.

Today her secrets are ours. Not only men but women as well—perhaps women especially at this point in time—have access to her wisdom. But today, rather than seek power *over* nature, we understand true realization as a process of harmonization *with* nature. This is an enlightenment that can only be attained when we fully and consciously come to inhabit our bodies. When we do this, we can live even better than the gods. Perhaps that is why it is said in India that the gods envy human beings—because it is only with a physical body that we can live out and outlive our karma and finally attain true wisdom. Higher than the gods, then, is the state of the yogi and yogini. Through yoga we realize transcendence without losing our humanity. With this knowledge, we can transform the world.

It is in nature that we find spirit in its purest manifest form. Nature teaches us the most about who we are, not through thought but on the deeper level of resonance. Nature reflects our most primal reality back to us: that at the most basic level we are made of the same elements as the earth. While science observes the laws of nature in order to predict and control, the yogini resonates with nature in order to surrender to its most basic and universal principles. The larger patterns of the universe can ultimately not be totally grasped with the limited mind. The mind can in the final analysis only be a jumping-off point for cosmic consciousness, an apprehension of Universal Being with the total human organism.

Understanding this well, holy men and women in India are usually found living in natural settings, in mountains or caves, near waterfalls and rivers where they can contemplate nature in undivided unity: inner nature reflecting the outer. Likewise, nature should be a part of our own yoga practice. If we are receptive, nature has the power to balance and humble us, to teach us to view ourselves within a larger context and to maintain a healthy and respectful relationship with other species, both animal and plant.

Why do some yogis subject themselves to extreme heat and cold, sitting by fires in the dead of summer and bathing in icy rivers in winter? I suspect it is for the same reasons some of us in the West enjoy wilderness camping. By exposing ourselves to the weather, we not only test our limits, where our bodies end and the environment begins, but we also come to understand on increasingly subtle levels how much we are influenced by larger forces in the universe. Whether or not we are consciously aware of it, the earth responds to the moon and the sun and other cosmic rays and, as a part of that earth, so do our bodies. To resonate with nature involves all five senses, and other more subtle sensibilities of which we as a species are not yet, or are no longer, aware. But to tune in to these processes we must give our minds a rest and open our inner as well as outer senses, to turn off culture, which invariably involves some kind of activity, some kind of doing, and tune in to nature, which allows us simply to *be*.

The Dance of Nature

Yoga is "elementary." From the yogic viewpoint, the most basic level on which nature can be both experienced and conceptualized is that of the panchabhuta, or five elements: earth, water, fire, air, and space. These interact in an infinite number of permutations and combinations to make up creation, the yogini's mirror. Nature reflects the yogini's dance, which displays both set patterns and spontaneous joy and innovation. Through conscious meditation on these elements we too can identify our physical body with its constituent elements, to totally merge with the environment, to identify with the forces of nature and thereby free ourselves from the limitations of our physical reality. In this way the realm of the natural moves into that of the psychic or the "super-natural," for, more than material substances, the panchabhuta are also abstract principles or qualities with metaphoric and spiritual significance, principles for understanding the human body, mind, and consciousness as well as the manifest universe.

This is reflected in the five elements, which in tantra are mapped on the human body in the various chakras. Earth is visualized as located in the muladhara chakra, located between the anus and the sexual organs. Water is located in the svadisthana chakra, located in women in the yoni or vulva/vagina and in men at the base of the penis. Fire is located in the manipura chakra, which is both the digestive center and the center of will in both men and women. Air is located at the heart center, the anahata chakra, and space is located at the throat center, the vishuddha chakra. In turn, each of these chakras and elements is related to a corresponding sense, which are all in fact only truly experienced in the head, in the brain centers and their immediate sensory extensions: earth, or muladhara chakra, is associated with smell, whose sense organ is the nose; water, or svadisthana chakra, with taste and the tongue; fire, or manipura chakra, with sight and the eyes; air, or anahata chakra, with touch and the lips; and space, vishuddha chakra, with sound and the ears. The head or skull, the area of the human body above the neck, mirrors the body—the five chakras that exist below. The elements are thus experienced both on the immanent level of unmediated nature, or instinct, in the body, and on the more abstract, transcendent level of culture, or conceptualization, in the head. Another way of putting it is to use an electrical metaphor: while the switches exist below the neck, in the body, the lights actually go on inside the mind. While we directly experience the world through our senses, our understanding of that experience, our self-conscious awareness, is the function of our psyche, represented by the higher chakras.

These chakras are located in the head region, beginning with the ajna, located in the forehead between the eyebrows, the chakra of time, also known as the third eye. Some systems of yoga teach that this chakra is related on the physiological level to the pineal or the "master gland" located in the center of the brain. Modern science is only now beginning to research and understand the function of this gland, which is related to the regulation of all the other glandular systems in the body. The ajna chakra is also related to the eyes and corresponds to the sensation of sight, but in the Indian system there are three eyes. The right eye represents the past and the left eye the future; the third eye represents the present, the intersection of past and future as well as the transcendence of these two concepts in the eternal Now. Once the third eye is opened the past and future fall away. One is able to live fully in the moment, in the realization that there is really no such thing as time, there is only awareness of movement, of process, which gives rise to the concept of time as an independent construct. In meditation or yogic states of consciousness, as long as you are still perceiving form or movement you remain within the confines of time and have not yet moved beyond the ajna chakra.

The highest level within the physical body is that of the sahasrara chakra. This chakra is located in the brain and represents the totality of the human organism, for everything that exists below is mapped there in the central nerve-command center. Your body can be in perfect order, but if there is damage in the brain you cannot function in the corresponding part of the body. There is a great deal of truth in the saying that the universe exists only in your mind, because without consciousness there would only be instinct, not perception or human experience as we understand and reflect upon it. What distinguishes humans from other animals, even primates, is basically the ability to reflect upon one's own actions, one's instincts, and the will to choose an appropriate response in the gap that exists between the instinctual trigger and the time it takes to act upon it. This is the essence of the human moral capacity, which has given rise to culture. It is that which uniquely defines humanity, the transcendent impulse that enables the human to rise above the instinctual level of "raw" nature and survival.

The sahasrara is visualized as a thousand-petaled lotus that sits on top of the spinal cord like a lotus on a long lotus stalk, an exquisitely complex and fine-tuned step-down transformer capable of channeling vast cosmic energy into the unique and limited form that creates you or me. It is a delicate balancing act that is made possible only by the support of the body, the physical frame. Hence, all the more reason to respect our bodies and their processes. In tantra the final goal is visualized as a union of all parts of the self, between the "lower" and "higher" human capacities, between all the elements and their abstract alchemical properties, between the senses and the one who is sensing, the seer and the seen. This is understood as a process akin to sexual union, in which the female

Kundalini or individualized creative energy that lies coiled in the muladhara chakra at the base of the spine is aroused and, in a movement that both mirrors and reverses creation, rises to the uppermost chakra, the sahasrara, which is conceived as passive male awareness. There the female energy of Kundalini unites with the male energy of the sahasrara. The mating of instinct and awareness, of creation and transcendence, of the individual ego and Universal Being, is the goal of tantra, and is the ultimate spiritual realization. When this happens, the eighth chakra appears as the universe itself, conceived as all that is beyond the boundaries of the body but with which the body is in constant communion. The eighth chakra stands for harmony with the entire universe. At this level there is no distinction between self and the world. There are no boundaries, no limits. The self has become infinite. We are one with the universe.

But what if we are not ready to reach that state? It is presumptuous for us to think that simply because we can conceive of this process we are capable of achieving it. Nonetheless, once we know that such a state exists, it changes our lives forever. For the first time we are aware of our own limitations, and something in us will not finally rest forever in ignorance. At least on the conceptual level we can understand the nature of existence and begin to strive for wisdom and compassion, for health, peace, and the joy that is the antidote to the suffering that limited existence necessarily involves. We can commit ourselves to the respect and protection of nature, both within us and without.

Merging *back into* nature, we identify our bodies with the elements, that dissolution itself a process of transcendence. We may not be ready to become gods, but we can gaze into the yogini's mirror and come to understand her teaching: We are all of the above, and all below. All is becoming. We are the becoming.

The Yogini's Dance: Dance of the Panchabhuta

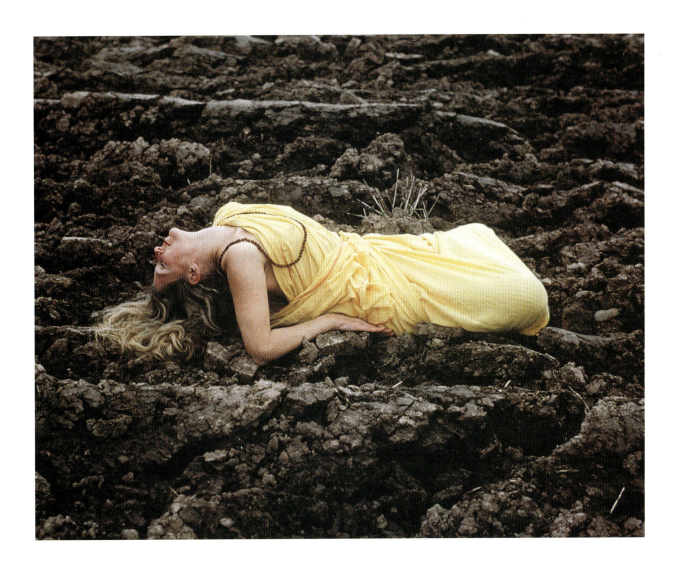

❧

I feel myself become earth, the solidity of form and weight of permanence. My body merges into the full materiality of clay, rock, and soil. I am density, heaviness, substance. I am stability and endurance to withstand the ravages of time. Water washes over me, seeps into me, softens me; fire burns on me, air envelopes me; space gives birth to me. I am earth.

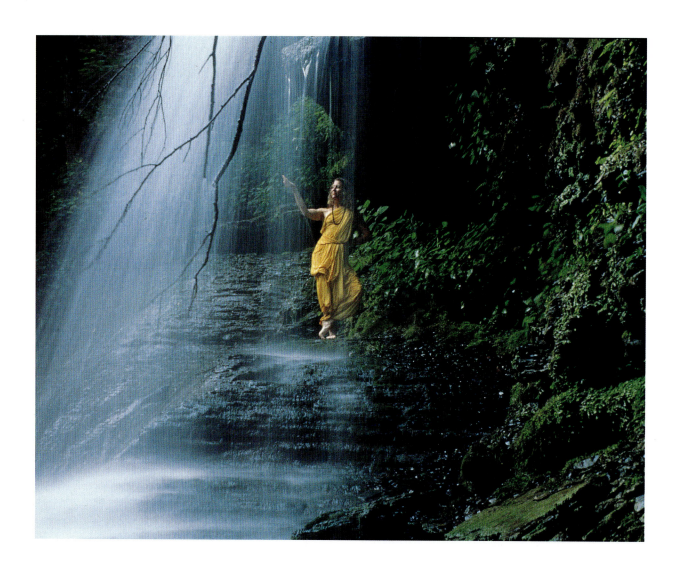

※

I feel myself become water, the primordial fluids of life. My body spreads over all the earth to give birth to all living plants and animals. Rising and falling with the moon and sun, I renew, replenish, and purify all that breathes. Following the path of least resistance, I wash over vast landscapes toward my ultimate resting place—the sea—becoming the vast and peaceful ocean of bliss. I flow over earth. I quench fire. I purify air. I mirror space.

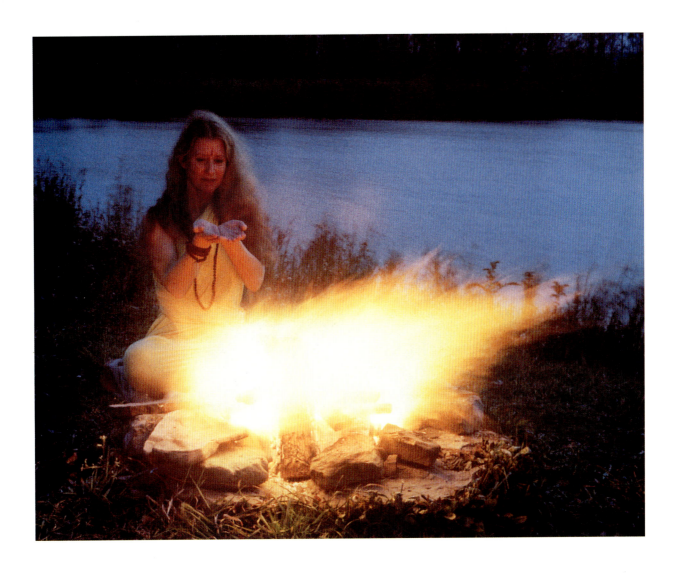

❧

I feel myself become fire, the raging power of transformation. I rise like smoke from the smoldering embers of sunset, strike like lightning in the dark night. In dancing flames I lick the sky, reduce all solidity to ash, offer all substance as sacrifice to the ten directions. I consume earth; I turn water into vapor. I feed on air. I fill space with light. I am fire.

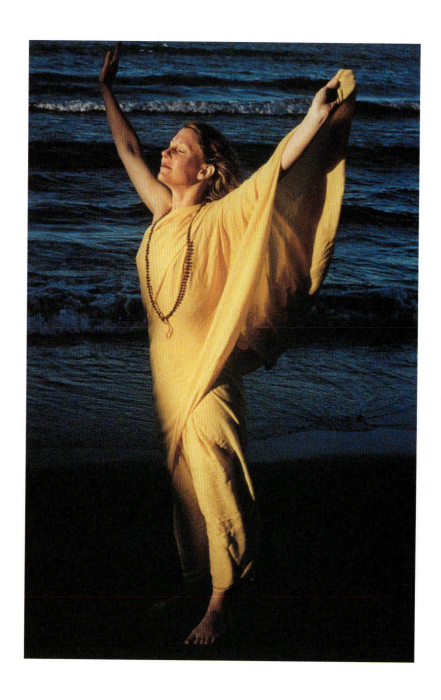

❦

I feel myself become air, the spirit that moves over the earth and in all creatures as the breath of life. As wind I move through trees, rise to mountaintops, traverse rivers and valleys, and rage at will, churning deserts and oceans. I can be as invisible as the night sky, or reveal myself in sun-streamed silver clouds. The most subtle of all substances, I am the father of life itself. I sustain the earth. I churn the waters. I feed all fires. I move through space. I am air.

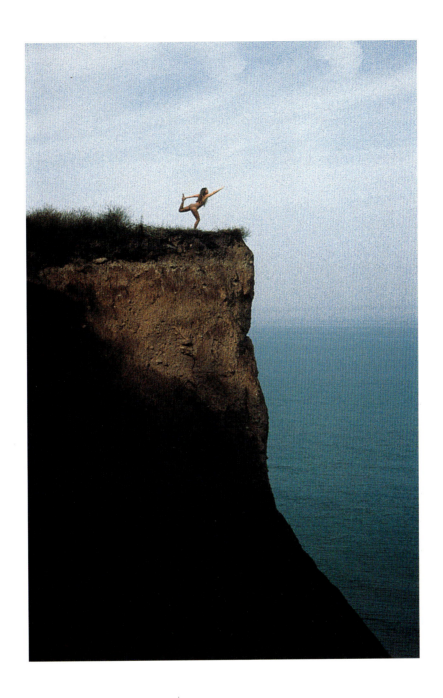

❈

I feel myself become space; the ten directions; depth and span; the cosmos; Akash, the infinite sky; and Sunya, the absence that makes presence possible. I manifest as expansion and containment, the cosmos as womb, Mother of the Universe, the beginning and the end of time. I am distance and proximity, that which exists between all other elements. I am fullness. I am emptiness. I am the circumference and I am the center. I am space.

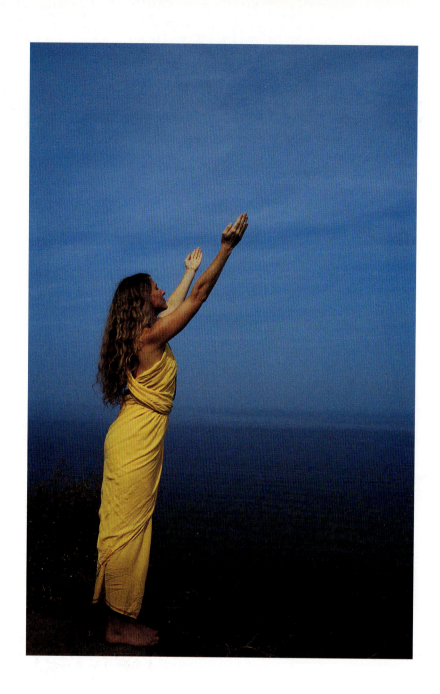

❧

I am the five elements and in me they are one. I am their infinite dance, the play of substance and form, nature and culture. I am the male and the female, the ideal and the real, locked in infinite embrace. I am the movement and the stillness at the center, the darkness and the flickering light. I am the origin and the never-finished end. I am divine detachment and intimate human compassion, witness consciousness and willful, blissful ignorance. I am Supreme Awareness, the lamp and the flame.

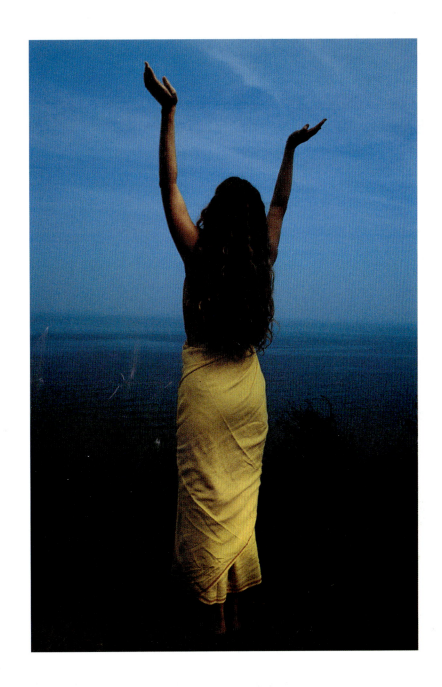

❦

I am the yogini and the mirror's reflection. I am the dancer and I am the dance.

Bibliography

Archer, W. G. *The Loves of Krishna in Indian Painting and Poetry*. New York: Grove Press, 1957.

Bharati, Agehananda. *The Ochre Robe*. 2d ed. Santa Barbara: Ross Erikson Publishers, 1980.

———. *The Tantric Tradition*. London: Rider & Co., 1965; Garden City, N.Y.: Doubleday, 1970.

Coomaraswamy, Ananda K. *The Dance of Siva*. N.p.: Asia Publishing House, 1948.

Dehejia, Vidya. *Yogini: Cult and Temples*. New Delhi: National Museum, 1986.

Gupta, Roxanne Poormon. "The Politics of Heterodoxy and the Kina Rami Ascetics of Banaras." Ph.D. diss., Syracuse University, 1993. Abstract in *Dissertation Abstracts International* 5408, no. 9401681 (1993) 3087.

Haberman, David L. *Acting As a Way of Salvation: A Study of Raganuga Bhakti Sadhana*. New York: Oxford University Press, 1988.

Kersenboom-Story, Saskia C. *Nityasumangali: Devadasi Tradition in South India*. Delhi: Motilal Banarsidass, 1987.

Khokar, Mohan. *Traditions of Indian Classical Dance*. 2d rev. ed. New Delhi: Sangeet Natak Akademi, 1984.

Marglin, Frederique Apffel. *Wives of the God-King*. New York: Oxford University Press, 1985.

Ramachandra Rao, S. K. *Sri Chakra*. Delhi: Sri Satguru Publications, 1989.

Tigunait, Pandit Rajmani. *Sakti Sadhana: Steps to Samadhi*. Honesdale, Pa.: Himalayan Institute, 1993.

van der Veer, Peter. *Gods on Earth: The Management of Religious Experience and Identity in a North Indian Pilgrimage Centre*. London: The Althone Press, London School of Economics, 1988.

Vatsyayan, Kapila. *Classical Indian Dance in Literature and the Arts*. New Delhi: Sangeet Natak Akademi, 1968.

White, David Gordon. *The Alchemical Body: Siddha Traditions in Medieval India*. Chicago: University of Chicago Press, 1996.

Wilbur, Ken. *A Brief History of Everything*. Boston: Shambala, 1996.